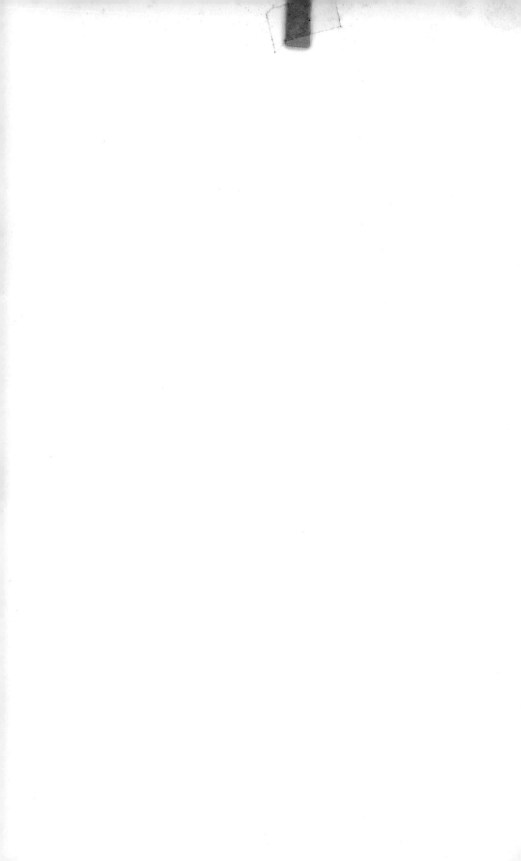

THE FUNDAMENTAL IDEAS OF MEDICINE

A Brief History of Medicine

A Monograph in
THE CARL VERNON WELLER LECTURE SERIES

Edited by
S. E. GOULD, M.D.
Professor of Pathology
Wayne State University College of Medicine
Detroit, Michigan

THE FUNDAMENTAL
IDEAS OF MEDICINE

A Brief History of Medicine

By

J. F. A. McMANUS, M. D.

Professor of Pathology
The Experimental Program of Medical Education
Indiana University
Bloomington, Indiana

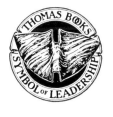

CHARLES C THOMAS • PUBLISHER
Springfield • Illinois • U. S. A.

Published and Distributed Throughout the World by

CHARLES C THOMAS · PUBLISHER

BANNERSTONE HOUSE

301-327 East Lawrence Avenue, Springfield, Illinois, U.S.A.

© 1963, by CHARLES C THOMAS · PUBLISHER

Library of Congress Catalog Card Number: 63-15428

*With THOMAS BOOKS careful attention is given to all details of
manufacturing and design. It is the Publisher's desire to present books
that are satisfactory as to their physical qualities and artistic possibilities
and appropriate for their particular use. THOMAS BOOKS will be true
to those laws of quality that assure a good name and good will.*

Printed in the United States of America

P-4

Preface

HIS BOOK describes the historical development of the fundamental ideas of medicine, i.e., the presuppositions on which medicine is based, the ideas that have made modern medicine. For example, physicians believe that the patient and his disease can be studied intelligently and in many instances treated adequately. How these ideas have originated, many in the ancient world, and matured over the course of centuries so that they are now accepted and taken for granted, is recounted briefly.

This is in a real sense an outline of the History of Medicine, presented in an abbreviated and more readily absorbable form. The usual standard textbooks which deal with the history of medicine are large compendiums devoting a considerable amount of their space to the lives of the great workers in the field. The more important aspect, the ideas which these outstanding people proposed or opposed, tends to be submerged in the voluminous life histories of the great and near-great. The present book describes the fundamental ideas of medicine with only a moderate attention to their proponents or antagonists, not because the men were not important but because the ideas are even more important.

Brief biographic notes on over one hundred fifty of the individuals named in the chapters are included and arranged alphabetically in the Appendix. Emphasis has been placed on details related to science and to medicine. It is hoped that these notes may satisfy the curiosity of the busy student or doctor who has no great amount of time to recall or to learn something about the great figures in science. Others, more fortunate in available time, may be stimulated to read further among the volumes and journals listed in the References.

Such a book as this must be derivative out of necessity, and must depend on the work of many scholars and on published articles and books. Because of the volume of material reviewed, I have not referred specifically to even a majority of the articles or books consulted. In the references are given suggestions for further reading of key articles and books in which one can expect to find additional data.

The invitation from the Committee for the Carl Vernon Weller Lecture of the Michigan Pathological Society to deliver the 1962 Lecture gave me at the one time a stimulus to re-work notes and data which had been collected over a number of years and an opportunity to organize them into a summary presentation. I am grateful to the Committee and to its chairman Dr. S. E. Gould, both for the invitation and for an opportunity to pay my respects to Professor Carl Vernon Weller, the late Professor of Pathology, the University of Michigan, Ann Arbor.

I am grateful to Mrs. Harold Hoppe Jr. who has not only typed the manuscripts but has also been very helpful in many of the required library chores.

I am grateful to Mrs. Sarah Brown, Librarian, The University of Alabama Medical Center, Birmingham, for allowing me to use the portraits preceding all but two of the chapters and for the use of the Frontispiece portrait.

J. F. A. McMANUS

Bloomington, Indiana

Contents

THE FUNDAMENTAL IDEAS OF MEDICINE

A Brief History of Medicine

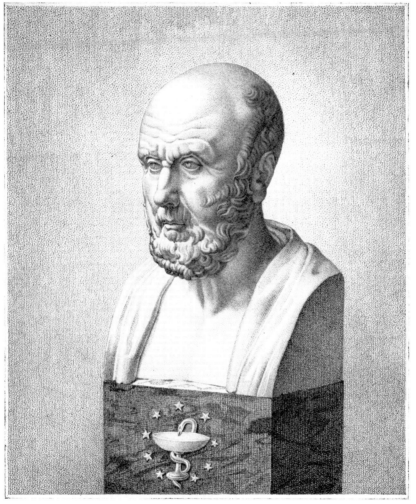

Frontispiece.

"The Father of Medicine"
Hippocrates of Cos
Portrait bust, not contemporary.

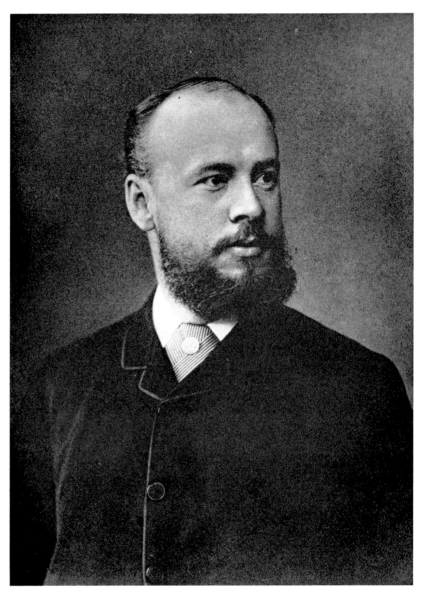

Welch (1850-1934)—Pathologist, Educator, Historian.

(From the Author's Collection.)

Chapter 1

Introduction—The Uses of History
The History of Medicine—The History of Ideas

HE STUDY of history has always been of interest to educated men. The great Aristotle regularly began his discussion of a particular aspect of his philosophic works with a historical review of what his predecessors had thought on it; so much was this evident in his works that his teacher, Plato, is reputed to have deprecatingly called him "the reader." Ever since then, reasonable men have realized that the currently prevalent ideas and the world as-it-is can best be understood in terms of the past which produced them.

Rowse has rightly pointed out that if each man had only the experience of his own lifetime, the span of three score years and ten which the Bible promised and which Science seems about to give us, about all any one man could learn would be a restricted knowledge in keeping with the shortness of his existence. With history, man can become one with the record of the human race; insofar as he has an acquaintance with history, man can profit from the experiences of all his predecessors.

Further, there is a definite cultural value to history, as Collingwood especially has emphasized. A professional philosopher, but by avocation and inclination a historian, Collingwood regarded one of the chief contributions of history to man to be Self-knowledge. History tells us what man has done and therefore what man is. Viewed historically, the past is revealed to be more than a series of episodes involving people in action; it is seen to be filled with struggle and adventure, as the world in which we live is gradually constructed by the strugglers, those who differed from and added to the times in which they lived. Muller speaks eloquently in this fashion of the use of history:

> "As has been said, one who knows only his own time and place cannot even know that. For the object is not only a better understanding of other peoples, humane and valuable though it is. It is finally a better understanding of ourselves; of who we are, and where we are and how we got this way; of both our achievements and our failures, our strength and our weakness."

It can be said, regarding Medicine, that one who knows only current information about Medicine does not know even that.

Many of our most eminent physicians have been enthusiastic and informed historians, followers of Clio Medica. Sir William Osler ranks perhaps highest among American physicians in transmitting his own interest in history to his pupils. His colleague at Hopkins, William Henry Welch, helped form the magnificent medical historical library in that institution and occupied its first Chair of the History of Medicine, since graced by Sigerist and by Shyrock, the former a Welch discovery and recruit. Other names among only the Americans interested in the history of medicine which come readily to mind include Harvey Cushing, John Fulton, Gross Harrison, Ralph Major, and William Bean. Many others, too numerous to name, while less distinguished scientifically, have similarily preached the usefulness of Medical History in improving our understanding of Medicine and even our Medicine itself.

We are fortunate in having a number of good textbooks in the history of medicine as well as several periodicals in which the fruits of historical research in medicine can be published and read. The textbooks of the History of Medicine, listed in the references appended to this book, include the classic work of Garrison, recently reprinted, the two volumes of Sigerist's series, unfortunately interrupted by his death, Major's two volumes and the same author's *Classic Descriptions of Disease*, Mettler's volume and Shyrock's, as well as Bettmann's *Pictorial History of Medicine* and Guthrie's textbook.

There is then no lack of suitable books as a good reason why a medical student or a physician should not be well acquainted with the history of his profession; his predecessors on the proud path which he is treading should be well known to him.

However, there is one limitation in this regard. It consists quite simply in the onrush of the development of new knowledge, the volume of which must tend to overpower the student and the practitioner alike. William Boyd in remarking on this, and noticing that medical literature seems to have reached the logarithmic phase of growth, aptly quotes *Alice Through the Looking Glass*, "it takes all the running you can do to keep in the same place. If you want to get somewhere else, you must run twice as fast as that." The competition for the time of the student and practitioner by his studies on the one hand and by practice on the other, combined with the formidable continual increase in essential knowledge makes it unlikely that a large volume of medical history will be read at all thoroughly. Its very size and completeness may act as a deterrent to any such reading, no matter how much it is desired and how valuable it is realized to be in many respects.

The solution may well have come in what Lovejoy has termed the History of Ideas. The heroes of medicine—the Vesaliuses, the Pares, the Hunters, the Virchows, the Billroths and the Halsteds— are important as the originators or as the protagonists or antagonists of Ideas which have dominated and directed the development of medicine. The study of the history of ideas in medicine may be regarded as showing in somewhat concentrated form the forces that have determined our present situation.

In a sense the history of ideas in medicine is broader than the history of medicine itself. The presuppositions and operative ideas upon which medical advance has been based are found in other provinces of thought and in different periods of time. The further development of the fundamental ideas in medicine which is presented in the remaining chapters in this book will help to make this clear but some preliminary additional comments are in order.

In the development of medicine as it is today, recognizable beginnings were made in antiquity by philosophers, by priests, by scientists and by others difficult to categorize because of their versatility, such as the mystic-mathematician-philosopher Pythagoras, or because of lack of precise knowledge about them. Later, the patterns of thought of the time, originating in fields at first glance far removed from practical medicine, greatly influenced medical thinking and subsequently, medical practice. In the following pages one can then expect to find names which were not initially connected with medicine but which will, I hope, be shown to have influenced our present status as physicians and probably our future hopes.

I must emphasize that the ideas presented as being fundamental to Medicine are those chosen by me. It is hoped and expected that, for other individuals, quite different ideas will appear of equal or greater importance. The ideas presented seem to me at this time as the most fundamental; they are the results of several years of special consideration of the ideas common to medicine and of many years of interest and study of medical history, an interesting hobby during my years as a student and teacher of pathology.

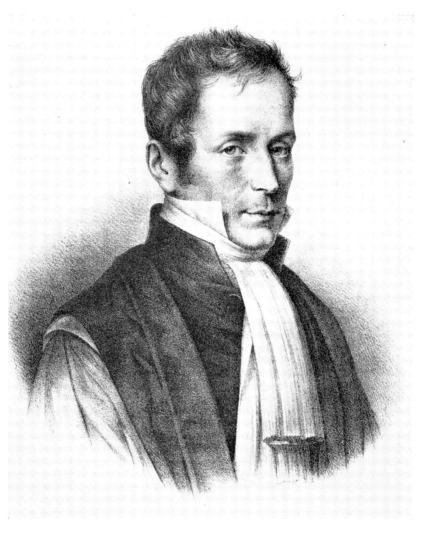

Laennec (1781-1826)—Father of Physical Diagnosis.

Chapter 2

Abnormal Conditions Can Be Recognized in the Living Body

F ONE were asked to select the single most important idea upon which medicine is based, I rather think it would be the one outlined in the title of this chapter; that abnormal conditions in the human body can be recognized. Corollary to this is the implication that the condition recognized as abnormal is in fact abnormal. I do not plan to enter into any complicated or lengthy discussion of the idea of the normal. It is generally agreed that the normal is the average, the usual, the everyday. The problems raised by the prevalence of "abnormality" in a population as, for examples, splenomegaly in children in malarious areas of Africa, or the former frequency of goiters in the inhabitants of the Alps or around the Great Lakes of North America, or by the recent discussions of the frequency (up to $70^+\%$) of mental "abnormality" in the dwellers in urban New York, are beside the point and will not be discussed further. Normality and abnormality are expressions of the frequency of a set of values in a sample, the normal being the more frequent, the abnormal the less frequent.

Like so many of our ideas and beliefs, the earliest expression of the idea of normal and abnormal is to be found in the urban civilizations which grew and flourished in Sumer in what is now called Mesopotamia. Sigerist has illustrations of animal livers, both normal and abnormal, used by priests in divination ceremonies during which future events were predicted according to the configurations found in the organs. The Sumerian civilization dates back three thousand years before Christ. By 2000 B.C. Sumer had been overthrown and replaced by Babylonia, one of whose great kings, Hammurabi, includes in his code of laws instructions concerning penalties for medical and surgical mistreatment. One can then conclude that, not only were abnormalities being recognized, but they were also being treated two thousand years before Christ.

The urban civilization of Egypt, like Sumer, founded in a fertile valley, this time the Nile, had medical papyri dating back to 2000 B.C. and quoting material from 2980 B.C. Abnormal conditions were recognized and treatment was prescribed, including medicines, surgery, prayers, amulets and sorcery. These early Egyptian medical remains reveal an appreciation of disease and a range of therapy considerably in advance of even the later Mesopotamian medical writings. History tells us that antiquity thought highly of Egyptian medical information, so that Egyptian physicians were in demand even in Roman times.

The diseased individual was a subject for special study in Greece well before the 5th century B.C. when Hippocrates of Cos collected a series of observations of patients into a number of volumes, several of which have survived to the present time. The Hippocratic school regarded medicine as an art or technique while the earlier Pythagoreans had regarded it as a theoretic science. Diagnosis of disease and prognosis were thought to be the high points of practice. The Hippocratic school is memorable not only for the intellectual and moral level of its writings, as evidenced in the Aphorisms and in the Hippocratic oath still taken by many doctors as they receive their diplomas, but also as proposing an early theory of the nature of disease which was to persist for two thousand years. This will be discussed later.

Alcmaeon of Croton, about the same time as Hippocrates, developed a concept of disease founded upon the opposites of Anaximander (c. 611-547 B.C.), while Empedocles of Sicily (c. 500-430 B.C.) proposed a theory about the origin of monsters, by this presumably meaning congenital abnormalities. These contributions of the Pythagorean school, along with the Hippocratic corpus, suffice to show that by the 5th cenutry B.C. the concept of disease was recognized. Actually, Plato (429-348 B.C.) in the *Timaeus* has a description and explanation of health and disease which reinforces this conclusion.

The recognition of disease states as abnormal continues nearly five thousand years after this concept was first propounded in Sumer and in Egypt. At first the physician had only his physical senses with which to recognize and to characterize abnormality. Only in the late eighteenth and early nineteenth centuries was the physician's hearing assisted by the percussion of Auenbrugger and the introduction of the stethoscope by Laennec. Later in the last century, the practical measurement of blood pressure became possible, and before the turn of the century, the x-ray was added. All of these were methods by which the abnormal could be recognized.

Chemical determinations of body fluids and products became possible by the rise of chemistry in the nineteenth century and this method, increasingly in use, has furnished another yardstick by which the normal is to be measured and the abnormal identified. The increasing use of chemical methods in diagnosis, i.e., the recognition of abnormality, sometimes places a strain upon the laboratory facilities of even the best equipped and staffed hospitals and clinical centers. Some important implications of "normal" body chemical values and their subtle gradation into the "abnormal" have been discussed by Williams in his *Biochemical Individuality*.

The best publicized and known of the recent recognitions of the abnormal forms of living things is to be found in the area of mental illness. The frank forms of insanity and mental disturbances and deteriorations have been identified as abnormalities almost since recorded history began, but in recent years there has been an increasing ability to recognize minor and less obvious disturbances of personality which affect deleteriously the capacity of the individual to serve as a useful member of society. In many instances it has been appreciated that these mental abnormalities are early stages of the more serious illnesses long recognized. In other cases minor disturbances which do not inevitably progress to serious mental illness but which nevertheless handicap their bearers, have been identified.

In practical medicine the first question which presents itself to the doctor when he sees a patient is this: "Is the patient sick?" i.e., is the patient abnormal enough to require treatment? Following this, the physician attempts to make a correct diagnosis, and subsequently to institute the appropriate treatment. The basic first step can then be regarded as the appreciation of abnormality and this step is still the most important one, some five thousand years after medicine began.

It seems to me interesting that we are still recognizing abnormalities, not only in the field of mental disease just mentioned, but also in chemical values in body fluids and products, as well as in other areas. As the increasingly subtle and numerous techniques of modern science are applied to the study of the human being, it is probable that a better understanding of the normal and the more efficient comprehension of the abnormal will prevail.

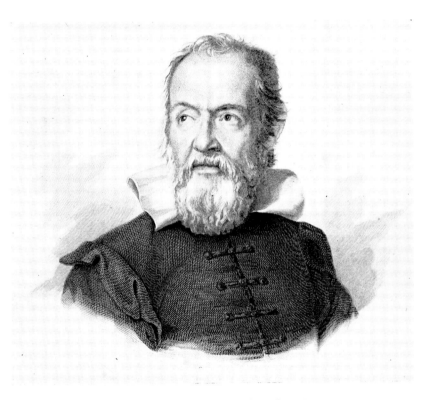

Galileo (1564-1642)—Maker of Modern Science.

(Courtesy of the Medical Library, the University of Alabama Medical Center, Birmingham.)

Chapter 3

The Living Organism Shares with the Rest of Nature the Properties of Being Orderly, Understandable and Analyzable

THE PRESUMPTION which is implied in the title of this chapter which says in essence that the living organism shares with the rest of nature the properties of being orderly, comprehensible and open to study, is fundamental to medicine and indeed to all science. If we did not have in our intellectual furniture the confidence in our ability to study and eventually to understand the living thing, and this means particularily understanding of the human being by the physician, we would surely not attempt to examine nor to treat the ill person. The idea is so basic that it seems quite obvious, but a momentary reflection will show that this is not so.

For our earliest ancestors, the world was one full of wonder and only poorly understood, and it remains so for the surviving primitive groups scattered around the world. Everything is alive, in the sense of possessing a spirit or soul, not only other men and all animals and plants but also such things as the stone and the soil and the rivers, and most especially the forces of nature, the storms, the wind, the rain, thunder and lightning. Over these "spiritual" forces man has no command nor can he comprehend the illnesses which characterize his own life. These must be caused by spirits; perhaps they are inimical to him, perhaps he has offended them. This view of the world and of himself man had in his more primitive stages, as history tells us and as is confirmed by our study of contemporary primitive peoples.

The beginnings of science can be found in the great valley civilizations of the Tigris-Euphrates and of the Nile, that is, in Mesopotamia and in Egypt. Mathematics probably developed as an aid to mensuration of the land which had to be re-surveyed after the periodic floods which inundated it. The floods conferred on the land a fertility which allowed the growth of the urban conglomerations in which the beginnings of law, medicine, science, art and business are to be found. Astronomy developed also in Mesopotamia and in Egypt, observations of the stars being used to assist in the measurement of time which depended primarily on the sun and on the moon. The development of both mathematics and astronomy in Egypt and in the Empires of Mesopotamia— Sumer, Babylon and Chaldea—was considerable from any viewpoint, being somewhat more advanced in Mesopotamia where a not inconsiderable application of mathematical methods to astronomical problems is found. That the Chaldean Astronomy degenerated into Astrology, in which it is believed that the stars influence the affairs of man and that events can be predicted from a study of the stars, should not detract from the considerable accomplishments of Mesopotamia which Neugebauer has pointed out.

Despite a degree of precision in mathematics and in astronomy, the beginnings of science in Mesopotamia can not as such be regarded as science as we understand it today. The first truly scientific works are to be found in Greece and her colonies, initially in Ionia. Here appears, for the first time, speculation on the nature of the fundamental substance of matter. That Thales in the 6th century B.C. suggested that everything in the world was made of water should not seem ludicrous to us. The important point is that man tried for the first time to explain the sensible world without the invocation of any spiritual elements and completely on a material basis with the fundamental substance familiar to all. Other later speculations included air, earth and fire as primary materials, while Democritus suggested that all matter was made up of minute and indivisible particles, atoms as he called them, foreshadowing our recent theories of matter.

Pythagoras, the founder of a brotherhood in a Greek colony in Italy, emphasized the importance of numbers to some of which he gave a mystic value. He also discovered the basic principle of harmonics in the relation between the length of a cord and the tone it produced. By his stressing the importance of numerical relationships as well as that of matter, Pythagoras gave a new additional dimension to things, a view still reflected in our chemical and structural formulae among other things. His school produced many notable scientist-philosophers, one of whom was Heraclitus whose statement, "One can never step into the same river twice," is by general consent one of the earliest statements of the essential change and flux which are observable in all things.

The beginnings of science as recognizable in the early Greek philosophers were rejected by Socrates (469-399 B.C.) who saw little value in such speculations when man, in his view, should be attempting to perfect himself. This, according to Socrates, who should rank as one of the first of the anti-scientists, man could do only by finding out what his purpose was in life. However, Plato, the pupil of Socrates returned to the consideration of nature in his systematization of knowledge. Plato was influenced by Pythagorean teachings to believe that the sphere was the perfect shape, and since the sun, the moon and the stars were the abodes of the gods, they must move in a circular course about the earth which was the central point in the universe. The spherical courses of the sun, moon and stars were mathematized by Plato's pupil Eudoxus (409-356 B.C.) and transformed into transparent crystalline spheres by Aristotle (384-322 B.C.).

By general agreement Aristotle is one of the great scientists of antiquity, so it is obvious that his reputation does not depend on his concept of world structure, although he remained best known for this for many centuries. Aristotle dissected and described a great many animals and studied the development of the chick from the earliest visible stage, by these activities replacing the speculation of the earlier Greeks with empirical observation. He was not above speculation himself and produced a theoretical mechanics which was to prevail for centuries as the explanation for the movement of objects. Certain prime materials, earth and water, had gravity and tended to move to the center of the earth, while the two others—fire and air—had levity and tended to flee from the center of the earth. All matter was made up of these four materials in various proportions.

Hellenic civilization moved to Alexandria upon the foundation of that city in Egypt by Alexander the Great in 322 B.C. as part of his plan to make the world Greek in culture and in knowledge. The great center of learning there was the Museum, a sort of early university with laboratories and classrooms and most notably the largest library until relatively recent times. Supervised in its beginning years by a pupil of Theophrastus, who was Aristotle's best and favorite pupil, the museum was the site of conspicuous progress in many areas of science and in mathematics. In Alexandria, Euclid the mathematician, Archimedes the mathematician and engineer, Ptolemy the astronomer, and many other scientists, including the first geographers, studied and flourished. Her medical school was noteworthy. Alexandria represents the highest accomplishments of ancient science.

Following the decline and fall of the Roman Empire in the early centuries of the Christian era, scientific knowledge and thinking went into a long period of eclipse. All that remained were a few works of antiquity, of which the logical works of Aristotle were the most influential, and some works of the Fathers of the Church, of whom St. Augustine (354-430), with his Neoplatonism derived from Plato's disciples in Alexandria, deserves special mention. The barbarian nations occupying the territory of the Roman Empire were the raw material from which Western Civilization was to be formed. The Eastern remnants of the Empire, centered in Constantinople in Greece, survived until 1453. Effete and decadent, increasingly weakened, it contained a few scholars with some acquaintance and competency with classic Greek and its great works. In the West the monasteries were the refuges for learning, especially after the monks were set to the laborious task of copying by hand the manuscripts by which knowledge was preserved and transmitted. In Ireland, knowledge of classic Greek persisted in the Celts who had been driven out of Roman Gaul by the first onslaughts of the barbarians.

The nearly extinct, prostrate civilization that had once been the Roman Empire was revived and reborn slowly over a period of centuries, culminating in a series of renaissances beginning with that of Charlemagne in the 9th century. Bursts of intellectual activity in the 12th and in each of the later centuries up to the great one in Italy in the 15th were sparked apparently by the recovery or rediscovery of ancient learning, and influenced an educated minority largely within the ranks of the clergy. Despite the development of local languages in the emerging countries of western Europe, Latin remained the official language of the Church and its teaching to the clergy demanded the continuance of some forms of schools. From these modest centers of learning, related initially to the monasteries, later to the cathedrals and finally developing into universities, the ferment of new learning was to emerge. In these so-called Dark Ages, the Church acted as a reservoir and disseminator of knowledge while, through her, trans-mission of the legal genius of Rome was possible. The Church was the only institution bridging the period between the glory of Rome and its classic learning on the one hand and the new European countries on the other.

A characteristic variety of philosophy developed in the cathedral schools and universities of the Middle Ages at the close of the dark ages. These were the "schoolmen" often criticized for the subtlety of their logical exercises, especially in the period follow-ing the scientific revolution of the 16th century. It is only fair to point out that the mental achievements of those who made the revolution were gained in church schools, dominated intel-lectually by the Schoolmen. Whitehead said that it was by way of Scholastic philosophy that the idea of natural events as under-standable and analyzable reached the innovators of the Renais-sance. Further, Crombie has described not inconsiderable scien-tific accomplishments in the Middle Ages, foreshadowing the greater achievements of the succeeding periods.

Galileo Galilei (1564-1642) was a scientist and philosopher who pioneered the major feat of the Scientific Revolution; as Crombie describes it, "that of changing the conceptual framework in terms of which man investigated the natural world as a whole." With-out going into details, it can be said that after Galileo, motion was explained by momentum and impetus rather than on Aristotle's mechanics, and that the earth was no longer the center of the universe but only one of a very large number of similar planets and revolving about the central sun (a heliocentric universe was substituted for the geocentric one); and man acquired a new confidence in his ability to understand the world and, indeed, himself.

Aristotle's world system was discarded and, by this change of viewpoint, Galileo came into direct conflict with established beliefs including those within the Church. St. Augustine had said much the same as Galileo wrote in one of his letters, that the Bible teaches us "how to go to heaven and not how the heavens go," and St. Thomas Aquinas (1225-1274), one of the greatest of the Schoolmen, had pointed out that the geocentric hypothesis of Aristotle as transmitted by Ptolemy was only a theory and might be superseded. Despite this viewpoint, Galileo's teaching was taken to contradict literal interpretation of the Bible and he was forbidden to spread his beliefs further. Needless to say, for this is fundamental history, the subsequent studies of Kepler, Brahe and Newton demonstrated the acceptability of the Copernican hypothesis which Galileo had espoused. One is able to say that Galileo had advocates within the hierarchy of the Church at the time he was tried and sentenced, so that the judgment represents a victory of one group of disputants rather than a unanimous verdict.

Great scientific figures are numerous in the beginnings of the revolution of thought sparked by Galileo. Francis Bacon, Lord Verulam, sometime Lord Chancellor of England, dedicated his period of retirement to the promulgation of the fashions in which he believed the secrets of Nature were to be forced from her, and how man was to gain mastery over nature. Harvey was discovering the circulation of the blood, and a little later Isaac Newton was mathematizing the universe and discovering by the prism the component colors of light. Scientific studies flourished in England, in France, Germany and Italy; and further, the new discoveries in science were incorporated into an intellectual effervescence in which philosophy was re-examined.

René Descartes (1596-1650), who by the way had taken some medical courses and wrote a book on the fetus, was a prolific and articulate scientist-philosopher who attempted to remain within the Church while re-examining her fundamental beliefs. It has been pointed out that a period of thought is marked out by St. Augustine's "I think; therefore, God is" and Descarte's best known phrase, "I think; therefore, I am." Broad in his interests, Descartes wrote profusely about many things including vision, the philosophical requirements of the investigator and about many subjects in physiology, including the circulation of the blood as discovered and described by Harvey a little while before.

In consideration of the movement of the blood, Descartes proposed a type of thinking which was to be permanently important in scientific thought: the mechanistic viewpoint as it is now called. By analogy with the clocks then appearing in Europe, Descartes suggested that the workings of the body could be compared to a series of clock-like machines in action. Wiener has pointed out that subsequent thinkers have likened the workings of the body to types of machines known at the time, the steam engine after Descartes, the chemical reactions when chemistry became popular, and so on to electronic circuits and feed-back today. Nevertheless, the contribution to thinking about the living thing by Descartes was impressive and remains an original work of great fundamental importance.

The pupils of Descartes and those who followed his line of thinking were numerous and themselves effective in further emphasizing the value to science of the analogy to the machine. The physician, de La Mettrie (1709-1751), a disciple of Descartes, carried his master's thesis further in the book, *L'Homme Machine*, the title of the work revealing its viewpoint. Another follower and another physician, Baron von Holbach, carried the mechanistic viewpoint to the logical conclusion describing existence as only matter and motion, without any spiritual force, influence or presence being implicated or suggested. The world has no order and no purpose, only necessity, says Holbach, in a gloomy foretaste of our contemporary, Lord Russell.

Descartes and his mechanistic interpretation of vital activities represents a departure from the thinking about life by most of those who had preceded him. Some of the Atomists and their Epicurean derivatives had conceived of life as the motion of particles but their doctrines were not widely known and where known, were not accepted as true. The prevalent thinking up to the time of Descartes had regarded life as consisting of organized matter infused with a soul (or souls), the different levels of vegetable, animal and human life each having a different soul. Bodily activities were explained as soul acting upon the body; along came Descartes who was prepared to understand bodily activities as resembling the workings of a clock.

Galileo's new mechanics and new conspectus of the heavens, agreeing with the theory of Copernicus rather than with the older Ptolemaic hypothesis originating with Plato and Aristotle; the confirming astronomic studies of Brahe and Kepler; and the combination of mathematics and astronomy into the system of Newton gave strong foundation for the belief of Nature as orderly, understandable and analyzable. This same way of thinking applied to the living thing or organism by Descartes, following the work of Harvey and the older studies of Aristotle and the Alexandrian scientists, gave confidence to the burst of scientific investigations which followed, as methods and techniques became available. This conspectus has persisted in science to the present day and especially is this true in medicine.

It is of fundamental importance theoretically but of little practical moment that Newtonian mechanics has been overthrown by the observations which have necessitated Einstein's Theory of Relativity. We do not have the same confidence as some of our immediate predecessors that everything can be explained in machine terms in the organism, or even by its logical extension in chemical theory. Certainly we lack the unbounding confidence of the scientists of the 17th and 18th century who looked forward to the conquest of nature, as Stephens describes them, with *naïveté* and unfounded enthusiasm.

While agreeing that the analytic and empiric mechanistic viewpoints have been supremely useful in developing new knowledge in science, which has produced some control of the forces of the atom and put man on his way to the moon and the other planets, there remains a reservation or two among many physicians and a great many biologists. To the mechanistic viewpoint of the living thing all who study the living thing, man or mouse, give operational validity: It works.

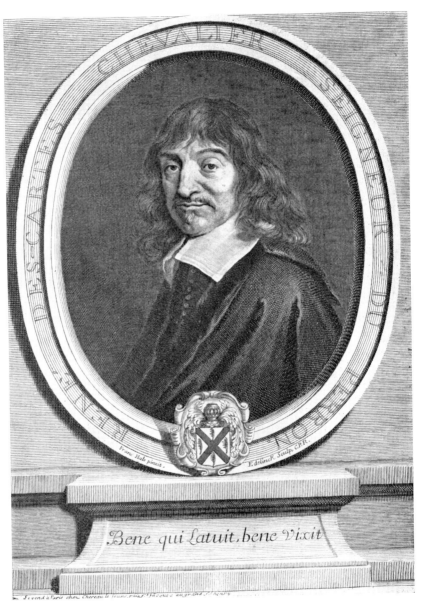

Descartes (1596-1650)—Mechanistic Physiology.

Chapter 4

The Living Organism Has Features of Structure and Function Which Can Be Examined Down to the Level of the Individual Cells and even to Subcellular Ultrastructure

HE STATEMENT at the beginning of this chapter will be appreciated as expressing the idea fundamental to the development alike of the study of structure in the anatomic disciplines and of the study of function in the physiologic sciences. Perhaps in none of the other fundamental ideas of medicine can the diverse influences of other intellectual disciplines be so readily related. The thinking about structure and function have gone hand in hand until relatively recently. As will be explained subsequently, there is continuing evidence that the present dichotomy is tending to disappear.

Aristotle (384-322 B.C.) is one of the greatest scientist-philosophers of antiquity. To Dante he was the "Master of Those Who Know," and in this century it has been said ". . . there is no main subject of philosophy or science on which he (Aristotle) has not said something still worth the hearing." His philosophy is the basis of the scholastic system of Aquinas which sparked the Renaissance of the 13th and 14th centuries and on which the makers of the scientific revolution were nurtured. Aristotle built a system which Cornford calls ". . . a colossal movement of rationalism, a compact and all-embracing structure furnished with an answer to every question." This systematic nature of Aristotle's work is at once a strength and a weakness, the latter because the followers of the

Stagirite tended to restrict inquiry and to neglect the very methods which were most valuable to him.

The biology of Aristotle is undoubtedly his major contribution to science. We have earlier seen that Aristotle's ideas on motion and the universe were both contradicted by Galileo, but the descriptions of several hundred animals which can be found in the surviving works of Aristotle have been very largely matched with surviving species. Dissections described reveal an interest in structure and an aptness in delineation of details which have delighted subsequent readers as diverse as Cuvier (1769-1832), one of the founders of comparative anatomy, and Charles Darwin (1809-1882), the father of the evolutionary theory. Separating living things from the non-living (although he seems to have believed in transitional stages between them), Aristotle had definite ideas on the relation between structure and function in the organism, as might be expected.

For Aristotle, shape (i.e., structure) is determined by function. Reverting to his own terms, "the form must be the cause in the sense of 'that for the sake of which,' " and, "If . . . artificial products are for the sake of an end (i.e., purpose), so clearly are the natural products." These statements of the structure of the part of an organism being determined by the purpose which the part serves are what is known as teleologic thinking, from the Greek *teles* = purpose and *logos* = knowledge. Many times the assumption that we can recognize a purpose is quite unjustified and the teleologic way of thought has been properly criticized. However, in everyday life we use terms in the Aristotlean teleologic sense, for example in the word "screwdriver." Similarily, in medicine when we talk about the circulation or the circulatory system to describe the cardiovascular system and the digestive system to denote the gastrointestinal tract, or when the surgeon asks for a clamp, or a hemostat, the spirit of Aristotle must smile in satisfaction.

You will notice that no mention has been given to any Sumerian or Egyptian contribution to the idea of structure and function. It may be that the appropriate records have not survived or that future translations of material may yet reveal some participation of the valley civilizations in the beginnings of anatomy and physiology. Despite the prevalent Egyptian ritual embalming, there is no evidence that any scientific study of structure took place. What suggestions there are of any appreciation of the function of a part are so imbedded in a matrix of magic and animism that interpretation beyond the mythologic becomes impossible or entirely a matter of speculation.

The Museum of Alexandria, already mentioned, was in a very real sense a memorial to Aristotle, for here was accomplished a combination of his biologic studies. From 300 to 288 B.C. Strato was its director; he was the pupil of Theophrastus, Aristotle's foremost pupil, and has been called the founder of Botany. Strato performed experiments on steam and the vacuum, and in neurology where he differentiated the sense organs from the mind and recognized that the mind formed sensations from stimuli. Herophilus, the eminent Alexandrian anatomist, is memorialized in *Torcular Herophili* where the venous sinuses combine posteriorly in the cranium. He also differentiated motor from sensory nerves and returned the seat of intelligence to the brain.

Erasistratus, a rival of Herophilus, described the heart valves in relatively good detail and traced the anatomy of the blood vessels as far as vision permitted. This anatomic study was supplemented by speculation on the function of the cardiovascular system. From postmortem studies he concluded that the arteries in the body contain only air and he explained the movement of the blood on Strato's vacuum studies. This theory was disproved by Galen (2nd century), the Roman physician who was one of the most prolific authors of antiquity. While Aristotle's major writings were lost or survived only in the unused libraries of Byzantium, and the Alexandrian anatomic studies were forgotten along with most of the scientific information which was discovered there, Galen's work survived into the middle ages, and through the Renaissance Galen was the most influential physician. Galen was still the yardstick to which any medical hypothesis or conclusion had to conform up until the Renaissance in Italy. Singer explains Galen's popularity on his espousing of the teleologic view of Aristotle which fitted well with the prevalent theologic world view of Christianity, but Albutt has described how good some of Galen's clinical descriptions and judgments turn out to be, when examined by a clinician.

Galen composed an anatomy which has survived until the present time and was the standard textbook of anatomy for centuries. Although human dissection, and possibly vivisection, had been known in Alexandria, Galen apparently dissected the Barbary apes, once prevalent around the Mediterranean but now found only in Gibraltar. These animals, and not man, served as the basis for the muscular origins and attachments in Galen's textbooks, as Vesalius later showed.

Galen demonstrated that the arteries contained blood during life and formed a scheme of the circulation of the blood which prevailed until the studies of Harvey in the 17th century. According to Galen, food ingested was taken by the portal vein to the liver where it received the *natural* spirit. The blood then traveled to the right side of the heart where the *vital* spirit was added, on circulation to the lungs, where impurities were cast off in breathing. Passing through pores in the interventricular septum, so small as to be invisible, the blood was forced around the body by the left ventricle. In the brain, the blood had the *animal* (from *anima*, soul) spirits added to it and it was then transmitted to the body generally by the nerves. This is a far cry from the operation of the circulatory system as we know it but served to explain the phenomena and this explanation was acceptable until a better theory was proposed by Harvey.

After Galen, no real scientific medical contributions arose in the ancient world. Orobasius, a Greek physician of the fourth century in Constantinople, was a great admirer and advocate of Galen and is credited with the establishment of Galen's pre-eminence as a physician. Whatever the reason, Galen's hundred and more books carried his erroneous anatomy and his false theory of the circulatory system into the Middle Ages and beyond.

With the breakdown of the Roman Empire and the emergence of the new nations in its western provinces of Europe, anatomy and physiology shared in the eclipse of all knowledge. Gradually the ancient works began to find their way back to supplement the false theories and descriptions of Galen and the more unreal material included in the other "scientific" books, the *Etymologies* of Isidore of Seville and the works of Livy and Pliny, preserved in fragments. The biologic works of Aristotle were translated in Sicily in 1235,

Later a Greek, Chrysoloras, was appointed to the Chair of Greek in the Florentine Academy in 1396. His knowledge of teaching of the classic Greek language and literature is regarded by Symonds as the major contribution to the great Renaissance, helped by the contributions of a number of Italians who had gone to Byzantium and had returned with a knowledge of and enthusiasm for classic Greek as well as with many manuscripts of the ancient authors.

Symonds, in his *Revival of Learning,* credits the Italian Renaissance of the fifteenth century on this application of Greek learning, science and criticism to the current problems. This movement became widespread in Italy and in 1447, during the Pontificate of Nicholas V, Rome is described as a vast workshop of knowledge, a sort of factory in which translations were made from Greek to Latin, the language of the educated of the time. Somewhat earlier the works of Aristotle on science, which had traveled with the Nestorian heretics from Greece to Syria before the 6th century and had been incorporated into Arabic learning, had been translated from Arabian to Latin in Spain where the tide of Islam had reached. The philosophic works of Aristotle, much admired by the Muslims, had helped to cause the earlier Renaissances, while the works of Natural Science were later arrivals.

Noteworthy in the medicine of the 16th century was Andreas Vesalius (1514-1564) who is properly called the Father of Anatomy. A native Fleming, Vesalius studied in Paris and taught Surgery at Padua after 1537. His great work, the *De Fabrica,* "on the structure of the body," was published in Basel six years later. The superb quality of his illustrations and the precision of the description of human anatomy raised anatomy to a new level and gave it scientific standing for the first time. While agreeing with Galen on the main course of the circulation of the blood, Vesalius raised some doubts about the "interventricular pores."

The 16th century is notable also for the work of Jean Fernel (1493-1558), delightfully memorialized by Sherrington, who introduced the term *Physiology* to describe the study of normal function as well as the term *Pathology* to describe the study of abnormal function. Immediately and universally accepted, Fernel's terminology of physiology and pathology for the study of the healthy and of the ill, respectively, is about as reasonable as dividing meteorology into separate disciplines dealing with good weather and bad weather.

Following Vesalius, anatomy developed as a science in its own right. Contributions to the knowledge of structure came from all over the European continent, notably Italy, France, Germany and Great Britain. The emerging discipline of biology began in the 17th and 18th centuries to notice features of structure in the lesser creatures which shared or could be conceived to share some of the features of human structure. Thus was born Comparative Anatomy, best represented in the studies of John Hunter of Scotland and Cuvier of France in the later years of the 18th century.

Long before this, the Englishman, William Harvey (1578-1657), had described the circulation of the blood from observations on living animals and by dissections. In studies at the great medical school of Padua, Harvey had learned the Galenic system but he had also observed the presence of valves in the veins. A number of years later, following computations of the volume of the heart and the amount of blood forced out of it by each beat, Harvey realized that the blood circulated around the body, the valves in the veins serving to prevent the blood from returning to the periphery instead of its usual path to the heart. From the right side of the heart the blood travels to the lungs and somehow passes through them to reach the left side of the heart where it is forced out to the body. How it got back into the veins was not clear to Harvey, but that it did was clear from the mathematics of the volume of blood circulated daily. Malpighi showed (1661) the existence of pulmonary capillaries by the use of the microscope and shortly other capillaries were demonstrated in other tissues. Harvey, with no better equipment than Galen had, managed to contradict Galen and develop a proper theory of the circulation. He did not dispense completely with the natural, vital and animal spirits of Galen and Aristotle, but relegated them to a place of secondary importance. Harvey, like Aristotle, studied the development of the chick embryo in the egg and contributed the first new knowledge on this subject since the ancient Greek philosopher, and published his studies in the book *On Generation* in 1651. But his fame correctly rests on his *de Motu Cordis*, "On the motion of the heart and blood," published in 1628.

Harvey's studies on the circulation rejoined the disciplines of anatomy and of physiology in the investigation of a single problem, setting a pattern which was to be followed for nearly two centuries. Stimulated by the success of Harvey's experimental approach and by the fashion in which Descartes propounded the concept that the living thing could be explained in machine terms, much advance was to be expected in the study of structure and function, but these hopes were delayed for a century and more by the absence of knowledge in the related disciplines which chemistry and microscopy were to supply. Above all, new instruments were needed and these took time to develop.

Embryology, as a study, developed and followed the lead of Aristotle and of Harvey but again it was handicapped by the lack of instruments, most specifically the microscope. In the interval before the microscope was perfected and auxiliary techniques developed, embryology became an area in which hypotheses flourished, one of which was to lead to the next great advance in biologic theory—the cellular theory.

It is customary to trace the origin of the cell theory to the animalicules which Leeuwenhoek (1632-1723) saw with the microscope, the small spaces which Hooke (1635-1703) saw in cork and finally the synthesis of Schleiden, Schwann and Dutrochet, which was applied by Virchow to the study of disease. In the history of ideas a different interpretation may be taken and this is the one which I will present.

Holbach, already mentioned in the discussion of Descartes' mechanism, synthesized his views into a work, *System of Nature*, which was published in 1770. This apotheosis of mechanism and the resultant logical materialism with no place for mind, soul or spirit caused a definite reaction in the German philosophers who were associates of Goethe, the scientist-poet-philosopher and universal genius. For the German philosophers the world of Holbach was inconceivable since the world was thought by them to be pervaded by a spiritual activity which resided also in every living thing. Schelling (1775-1854) was the leader of a group of Nature-philosophers who attempted a synthesis of a way of thinking dating back to Böhme (1575-1624) and Leibnitz (1646-1716), in which life was spiritual in essence, complicated in outline but notably anti-Cartesian and anti-mechanical. Life was the same in all things which were essentially self-developing individuals with self-contained structures. All living things were united also, said Oken (1779-1851), Schelling's associate, by being composed of, infusorial mucous vesicles, as he called them in 1805.

The promulgation of the derivative cell theory—that the structural unit of the living thing was the cell and originating in Oken's mucous vesicles—was accomplished by Schleiden (1804-81) for plants in 1838 and by Schwann (1810-82) in 1839 for all animals. Rudolf Virchow (1821-1902) had the pleasure of living until his cell theory of disease which he had described in 1858, and which stated that disease regularly consisted in disorder of the individual cells, had been accepted. Virchow stated further that cells come only from other cells, that there was no new formation of cells from anything except a pre-existing cell.

The general acceptance of the cell theory was followed by a series of studies which further detailed the finer structure of various types of cells. Initially depending on the recently developed achromatic lens systems assembled into microscopes, the later improvements in techniques involved the coloration or staining of tissue slices by natural dyestuff and then by derivatives of the aniline dyes first synthesized by Perkin in 1856. Thinness of the slices examined by the microscopes, microscopic sections as they are called, was made possible by the refinements of machine design and manufacture which the progress of technical ability made possible. In the confirmation and establishment of the cell theory we have then a good example of the fashion in which the various sciences react one upon another.

Improvements in microscope design with increasing magnifications to the limits of optical resolution have been followed by the invention in the 1940's of the electron microscope in which the light of the ordinary microscope is replaced by an electron source and the lens replaced by a system of magnetic fields. The resultant magnifications of the appearances of the cell structures have raised hopes that molecules may be visualized with further improvements in the optical system. Interestingly enough the preparation of tissues for the electron microscope and their study have involved many of the problems which were encountered when the light microscope was first used for the examination of tissues. Thinness appeared as a problem in electron microscopy as it had in light microscopy. The essential dilemma of seeking the "living" appearance in cells which have been "fixed" (i.e., killed) has not particularly perplexed electron microscopists.

Chemical methods of investigation began with Boyle in the 17th century and Lavoisier and Priestley in the 18th. Initially applied to the explanation of animal heat (i.e., metabolism) as it was called not so long ago, chemical methods were applied more and more to the study of animal structure and function. Purkinje, the anatomist-physiologist, opened the first laboratory for the study of physiology in 1824 and from then on the study of the organism by chemical methods has progressed at an increasing rate. The discipline first named Physiologic Chemistry is now generally known as Biochemistry.

The development of scientific physiology has been described by Goodfield in relation to the problems of respiration and animal heat. Following the formulation of its appropriate concepts, methods of inquiry and types of explanation deemed satisfactory, there was a period in which debate ensued concerning the appropriateness of physico-chemical methodology and experimental quantitative procedures. Claude Bernard (1812-1878) can be taken as the man in whom the viewpoints of modern physiology can be best recognized. His greatest contribution is in the idea of the constancy of the internal environment, the fluids of the blood and tissue spaces in which the cells actually live and function. The concept of constancy in the internal environment gave rise in time to the Homeostasis of Cannon, the tendency to stability or uniformity of the organism. It is noteworthy that Bernard related the structure to function in the following quotation:

> ". . . the internal environment created by an organism is special to each living thing . . . by its means (the physiologists and physicians) can act on the histological units which are the only effective agents in vital phenomena."

This relation of the internal environment to the cells which are the basic units of life in modern thinking is not always remembered by every physiologist.

With the multiplication of chemical techniques of various sorts and with the applications of diverse physical methods, the ultimate constituents of cells and tissues have been isolated and *en masse* subjected to sophisticated analyses. The current development of histochemistry and cytochemistry, by which chemical materials are identified within cells in microscopic sections, gives promise of putting back together and into an orderly picture of the cells the biochemical data which have been obtained by cell fractionation. Even more recent, the attempted application of cytochemistry to electron microscopy gives great promise, once the technical details and difficulties have been mastered.

Studies on living animals with radioisotopes have shown an impermanency—a turnover—even in what seemed to be the most stable structures, the teeth, the bone matrix and collagen, and at a more rapid rate in actively functioning cells and tissues. This recalls the idea of change and flux of Heraclitus mentioned earlier. Moreover the turnover studies suggest that both structure and function can be described in terms of process—process meaning a series of changes. As von Bertalanffy suggests, structure can be regarded as a process of long duration and slow rate while function is a rapid process of brief duration. (The "blow dealt to morphology" by Hume's idea of process has been recalled by Whitehead.) In terms of process, structure and function become one thing. Further, structure and function are back together as they were for Aristotle, for Harvey and for many other scientists of repute and accomplishment.

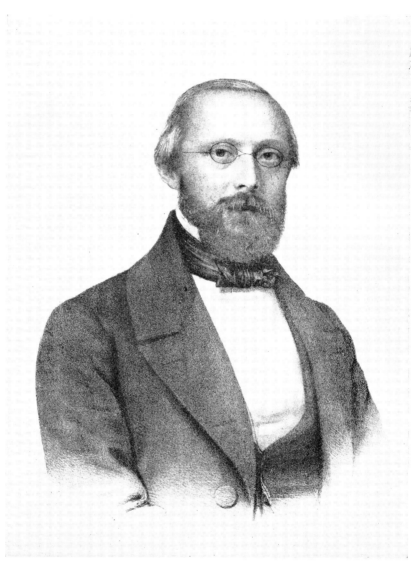

Virchow (1821-1902)—Modern Pathology.

Chapter 5

Disease Is an Alteration of the Body, Involving Both Structure and Function, even of Its Ultimate Units, the Molecules

BASIC IDEA currently prevalent in modern medicine, not always observed in the practice, is that disease is an alteration *of* the body, not something extraneous which is joined to the body during the illness. That this belief has not always been so general and that it is not held in all parts of the world even at the present time will be made clear in our subsequent discussion. We shall end this chapter by a description of the fashion in which the practicing medical man does *not* always behave in harmony with this belief, however obvious its truth may appear.

Our earliest ancestors believed that disease was caused by evil spirits or demons which had entered the body of the ill individual. The same notion of the nature of disease is held by many of our contemporary primitive peoples, the aborigines of Australia, the natives of Polynesia and, until recently, the American Indians. Various religious practices and rituals were, and are, performed to cure the illness and to do so by exorcising the evil spirit from the body of the sufferer. It has already been mentioned that the medical papyri from ancient Egypt of nearly two thousand years before Christ and dating back to sources nearly a thousand years older, included charms, amulets, and religious rituals in their therapeutic formulary.

In Ancient Egypt, as among our contemporary primitive societies, the physician is primarily a priest, as exemplified in certain parts of the African continent even today by the witch doctors with their strange costuming, charms, and practices, ritual dances and so on. In the Caribbean islands of the New World voodoo is still practiced among groups of the population, exotic ceremonies with an African past are practiced to cure, to cause or to transfer evil spirits which can cause harm and disease. A thriving business is done in a few cities of the United States, and in some other places around the world, trafficking in various unusual materials which are supposed by their ignorant purchasers to be able to ward off, or to cause, disease. Superstition these practices actually are, and can be properly called; their presence in current societies is nothing less than the remnant of beliefs held long ago in the presently civilized societies.

Hipprocrates of Cos in the 5th century before the Christian era appears to have been the first physician whose surviving records indicate that he held disease was *of* the body and not something foreign added *to* the body. This dictum was given in specific relation to epilepsy, which was called the "Sacred Disease" because it was believed that it was caused by possession of the ill person by spirits or by Gods. Hippocrates said forthrightly, "As for this disease called divine, surely it has its nature and its causes, as have other diseases." The history of pathology and even of medicine can be regarded as an elaboration and proof of the teaching of Hippocrates.

The school of Hippocrates appears to be responsible for an early theory of the nature of disease, the so-called Humoral Theory, that it was caused by a maldistribution of the four humors or fluids of the body. When blood is allowed to clot outside the body, four portions can be recognized in it: 1) a dark clot, 2) a red fluid, 3) the yellow serum, and 4) fibrin. Each of these was given a name related to a behavior pattern of the human being, and the behavior pattern was believed to be caused by an excess of one of the portions of the blood clot, while health was a proper balance of the four humors. With an excess of the dark clot material the patient was melancholic, with an excess of the red fluid the patient was termed sanguineous, the serum fraction in excess made the patient choleric, while an excess of fibrin produced a phlegmatic individual.

Several of these terms are still in everyday use, and persons are described as melancholic or phlegmatic. The humoral theory of disease was held in one form or another by physicians until the nineteenth century was halfway over.

Little concrete was done to determine the true nature of disease for over two thousand years, although much speculation can be found ranging from Plato in the *Timaeus*, wherein disease was described as a creature having a natural history, to the great Paracelsus (1493-1541), an alchemist and enthusiast who showed his disregard for the humoral theory by burning publicly the books of Avicenna in which it was described and from which it was taught as the revered authority. Aureolus Philippus Theophrastus Bombast von Hohenheim assumed the name Paracelsus to signify his own belief that he was superior to the ancient Celsus. This respected physician of Rome is still remembered for his cardinal signs of inflammation which are learned by all medical students, Rubor, Tumor, Calor, Dolor—Redness, Swelling, Heat and Pain. Paracelsus said that every disease is an organism, an individual, which is related to the body as the parasite is to the plant. Disease shows itself in different forms in different patients because of sex and individual differences. In each human being there is a ruler or *archeus* which maintains health, and during illness expels the disease and then returns health to the individual. In this statement there are hints of the Homeostasis of Cannon. Paracelsus said it was the duty of the physician in care of a patient to give the *archeus* an opportunity to exercise its healing influence.

The scientific study of disease can be said to have begun with the collection of autopsy reports on clinical cases by Benivieni and most notably by another Italian, Giovanni Battista Morgagni (1682-1771). In his *De Sedibus et Causis Morborum per Anatomen Indigatis* (On the seats and causes of disease as revealed by anatomy) published in 1761, Morgagni reported a large group of cases in which something of the clinical course and features are detailed and an attempt is made to relate these to the anatomic changes found in the individual on dissection. By his work, this anatomist can claim to be the founder of Pathology. As Payling Wright points out, that multifaceted genius Francis Bacon had suggested in 1605 in *The Advancement of Learning* that diseases should be examined by the dissection of cadavers and not passed over while the normal anatomy is studied, "whereas now, upon opening of the body they (the changes of disease—ed.) are passed over slightly and in silence."

Numerous autopsy data were gathered together in a systematic fashion according to organs by Matthew Baillie, John Hunter's nephew, in his *Morbid Anatomy of Some of the Most Important Parts of the Human Body*, published in 1795. Xavier Bichat (1771-1802) introduced the idea that disease existed in the tissues of the body, of which he had described twenty-one in 1797. This developing "tissue pathology" following on Baillie's "organ pathology" was halted by the premature death of Bichat, but Schwann's study of tissues which led to the cell theory has been related to his analysis of Bichat's descriptions. The application by Virchow of the cellular theory to the study of disease has already been recounted, culminating in the *Cellular Pathologie* of 1858. Since that time the existence of changes in the cells in all diseases has been presumed and in many instances has been proven.

The cellular pathology of Virchow temporarily vanquished the last citadel of humoral pathology (that disease was an alteration of the four humors of the body as suggested by Hippocrates in the 5th century B.C.) in the school in Vienna headed by Rokitansky. There were changes recognizable from the Hippocratic humors, terms such as Crasis and Dyscrasia had been added along with many others, but Rokitansky's teachings embodied the doctrine of the humors. In passing, the biochemistry, emerging about the time of the proposal of the cell theory of disease by Virchow and growing at a rapid rate, gave medical men another yardstick of disease and illness and eventually seemed to be a recrudescence of a Humoral Pathology as physicians began to treat the chemistry more than the patient.

From the cells of Virchow the lesions recognizable in the body constituents have now gone down to the level of the molecules. A molecular physiology had been predicted by Michael Foster in the 1880's and molecular disease was forecast by Gowland Hopkins and by Peters. A molecular lesion, that is a change caused by disease, has been recognized by Linus Pauling in the misplaced amino acid in sickle cell hemoglobin.

The idea of disease as having an existence separate from the body would seem to have been given the final quietus by the cellular theory of disease as described by Virchow and by the subsequent molecular defects found in a number of diseases. I would think that most physicians in North America would agree with this statement (although it has been mentioned by Rather that Virchow before his death regarded the disease as a separate entity —the ontologic theory), but practice is not always in keeping with belief.

The physician who treats the disease, or a sign, or a symptom, rather than the patient, or who treats the patient before a diagnosis is made, is acting as if the disease had a separate existence; he shares the ontologic theory of disease with the witch doctor and with Paracelsus. Similarily, the surgeon who talks about the "acute appendix he has" or the physician who talks about "the pneumonia he is treating" is acting on the same theory. The humoral theory reappears when the doctor treats the chemistry as an end in itself; most doctors have seen a patient who died in perfect "fluid balance" with the proper ionic values. Unfortunately the cells and the patient had died.

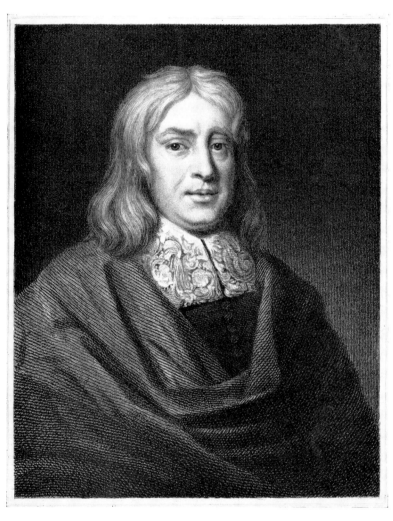

Sydenham (1624-1689)—Clinical Syndromes.

(Courtesy of the Medical Library, the University of Alabama Medical Center, Birmingham.)

Chapter 6

*Diseases Exist as Patterns of Bodily Processes
or Modifications of Both Structure and Function,
the Identification and Classification of Disease Processes
Extending Down to, and Depending upon,
the Molecules Constituting the Body*

T IS upon the basis of the beliefs that diseases exist as patterns of bodily processes and that they can be identified and classified that modern medical practice has been able to develop. If the diseases of the body existed in a random or haphazard fashion, and if they could not reasonably be compared one with another and sorted out, any attempt at diagnosis would be doomed to failure. And, further, if diagnosis were not possible then rational treatment also would be unlikely. A primary problem in medicine is, in this fashion, seen to be a biologic one: the issue of taxonomy which includes both identification and classification. We shall return to this aspect of things after tracing the fashion in which diagnosis has reached its present level of precision.

The medicine of Mesopotamia is known with regard to the practice of their physicians, and it seems to be largely a matter of incantations and ritual prayers along with some minor surgery and care of injuries. We are not quite sure about all of the diseases which were being treated by such methods although it does seem clear that cases of heart disease, eye disease, rheumatism, epilepsy and apoplexy were among those for whom physicians prescribed. Cataracts were known and couched as long as 2250 B.C. A disease

45

which has been thought to be leprosy is mentioned, its sufferers being cast out of the community permanently with an abjuration which says in part, "Never more shall he know the ways of his abiding place."

Much more is known of Egyptian medicine which seems to be considerably more advanced. This is in keeping with the high esteem with which Egyptian physicians were regarded in antiquity. Medical papyri—portions of which describe injuries, tumors, fractures, parasitic diseases, diseases of different parts of the body and the treatment thereof—are the chief sources of our information, although the travelers of antiquity have also given us some interesting data.

Herodotus tells us that the Egyptians had specialists, really a physician for each part of the body. He recounts that one doctor treated diseases of the eyes, another those of the head, another the teeth, and others the intestinal diseases and internal diseases. An interesting insight is given by the same traveler into the Egyptian's views on disease when he says the Egyptians purge themselves once a month for three days and preserve their health by emetics and enemas because they believe that all diseases come from food. While such practices may not have been unreasonable in Egypt where intestinal parasitic diseases were prevalent, one wonders how many centuries of intestinal havoc may have been wrought by these remarks since Herodotus follows them by comments on the healthy state of the majority of the Egyptians. It is a sad commentary on the low level of Babylonian medicine of the same time that Herodotus tells of the custom of bringing the sick person to the market place where the passers-by were expected and requested to tell of any acquaintance, personal or hearsay, with such a case and what treatment had been used.

The Greeks in history had three early groups of physicians, differing in their approach to disease. The oldest group was made up of the Asclepiadean, priests at the temples dedicated to Asclepius, the God of Medicine and son of Apollo. Aristotle the philosopher, the "Master of Those Who Know" to Dante, was the son of one of these. Another group was composed of Pythagoreans, followers of the mystic philosopher who is credited with founding mathematics. The third group was that of the followers of Hippocrates of Cos, who were earlier described as having originated the humoral theory of disease. While the Hippocratic group thought of medicine as both an art and a technique, the practical nature of their viewpoint being admirable to modern eyes, the Pythagoreans thought of the practice of medicine as an area for the construction of theory and for speculation.

Hippocrates is said by Garrison to have founded the bedside method, the close observation of and attention to the patient, which is the hallmark of the great physicians of succeeding centuries from Boerhaave and Sydenham to Heberden and Osler. The observational techniques of the Hippocratic physicians resulted in a meticulous and systematic examination of the patient's appearance, pulse, respiratory rate and type, bodily movements, excreta and sputum, and a careful inquiry after pain. A number of diseases have been recognized from the descriptions which have come to us as the Hippocratic corpus; among these are malaria, dysentery, depressions and mania, club foot, and tuberculosis of the spine which was associated with pulmonary tuberculosis. Observations on fractures and injuries of various sorts are included as well.

Various other schools of Medicine in the sense of sets of beliefs and techniques flourished in later Greece, in Alexandria and in Rome. Methodists, Pneumatists, Empiricists and others not worth mentioning, represent at the most, intellectual activity addressed to the problems of disease and variations of speculation resulting from the lack of sufficient fundamental information. This is not to say that clinical observation was not improved nor that the increasing volume of case histories did not allow the definition of more diseases. Hospitals existed in Rome in all probability and possibly also earlier in Alexandria. Celsus, apparently a plagiarist from the Greek Aufidius of Sicily, wrote on fever, on ascites, on anasarca, on tuberculosis, on apoplexy and on paralysis. Poisons receive a fairly lengthy treatment and human rabies following dog bite is described, as it was before then by Aristotle. Galen added clinical features of fevers and probably also some details of heart failure. Later Roman physicians added pneumonia, rickets, pleurisy, tetanus and asthma among many records, without distinction between symptoms, signs, causes, and the disease proper.

The medicine of antiquity bears the features which medicine was to show until the eighteenth and nineteenth centuries. The physician could inspect and palpate the patient, he could feel the patient's pulse and observe him carefully. He could recognize certain diseases conforming to his own experience or that of the limited number of medical works available, if he were fortunate enough to have access to them. To explain the disease state he had the humors of Hippocrates, the atoms of Democritus reappearing in the Methodist doctrine, or the *pneuma* of the Greeks in the Stoic-related Pneumatist doctrine.

Lacking any rational understanding of the body changes of disease, the physicians of antiquity were nevertheless remarkably successful in identifying individual diseases. However in many instances they believed that the signs and symptoms—fever, constipation, diarrhea, wasting, weakness—which are the manifestations of disease—were themselves diseases. In short, they were not able to distinguish in many instances between the disease and the body changes which resulted from it. This situation was to last for many centuries and many readers will recall Molly Malone of the song, who "died of a faver" (i.e., fever). More recent is the use of such terms as "dropsy" and "sore throat" for illnesses in which these body changes are produced by the disease.

With the decline and fall of the Western Roman Empire and during the period of development of the western nations out of the barbarian groups, the medicine of antiquity survived in Byzantium and later in Islam. Some diseases find good descriptions in the writings presently extant from these two centers, but no new ideas of consequence appear to have been added.

Medieval medicine (in the period from the 5th to the 13th century) shows few advances in the understanding of disease but many practical points of view appear which contributed to later advances. The growth under religious auspices of hospitals and of universities at which schools of medicine were instituted are two developments of the middle ages important in patient care and in the understanding of disease. A great deal of surgery was performed and recorded, really an amazing variety, and done with some understanding of asepsis as Crombie points out. Important in the development of surgery and its relegation to the barber-surgeons for subsequent centuries is the fact that the medieval church forbade its clerks to shed blood, thus closing the universities to the study and teaching of surgery. Crombie describes further the institution of the practice of quarantine in 1383 in Marseille to prevent the spread of disease by travelers, and an increasing interest during the middle ages in anatomy which was stimulated by the increasing surgical activity. Perhaps most important in the development of medicine, as Crombie points out, was the prevailing Christian theology with its emphasis on the value of the individual, the "charitable relief of suffering" and the "dignity" of labor.

The advance in science of the 15th and 16th centuries, culminating in the revolution of thought which flowered most exuberantly in the 17th century, gave many sorts of information and ways of thinking which were to be important in the historical development of medicine. However, it was in medicine that tradition was strongest. Ancient authorities like Hippocrates, Galen, and Celsus were well entrenched, and the new discoveries had to defeat the old theories before they were accepted. Bury, in his *Ideas of Progress,* has talked about the reverence for, and deference to, antiquity which was generally displayed until the 18th century when progress first was thought possible and, in fact, came into being. However, there were signs of stirring in the field of medicine and suggestions that the scientific advances of Galileo, Kepler, Newton and, in the biologic field, of Harvey, Malpighi and others, were not to be wasted.

The first task necessary in clinical medicine was the loss of theoretic explanations of disease by a return to the techniques of observation of the Hippocratic school. This was accomplished initially by Franciscus Sylvius (Franz de Boë), 1614-1672, who as professor of medicine at Leyden from 1658 until his death initiated the practice unique in Europe at the time, and for centuries before, of taking his medical students to the bedside. Here the patient was examined, questioned and his case discussed and the case was followed to cure or to examination by an autopsy if treatment was not successful. Another great professor at Leyden in the next century was Hermann Boerhaave (1668-1738) who was led into becoming a student of medicine and away from theology by the influence of his friend, the philosopher Spinoza. A skeptic about doctrines, a sympathetic, humane and kindly man, he generated an enthusiasm for the careful bedside study of the individual case which he transmitted to his students and they in turn to theirs. A man of broad education, his fame in time reached around the world so that he was sought as a consultant even in China. His place in medicine has tended to be somewhat reduced of late by critics. As Snapper points out, Boerhaave is the clinical teacher par excellence because of his own high qualities and because of his pupils who in Vienna, in Germany, in Scotland and then in England and the New England colonies, carried on the high standards he had established. Haller, the great physiologist, was one of his pupils and Cullen the founder of Clinical Medicine in Edinburgh was another, influencing the Hunters and through them Bright, while Benjamin Rush carried Cullen's methods, and through him Boerhaave's, to the Americas.

The sixteenth century, as well as seeing the rise of clinical teaching with Sylvius, also saw a reaction against any scientific emphasis in medicine. Early autopsy studies by Benivieni and Bonetti were neglected while Malpighi, remembered for his discovery of the renal glomerulus and of the capillaries which completed Harvey's circulation of the blood, was actually driven into retirement by ridicule and criticism. The father of microscopic anatomy was asked jeeringly what use was his microscope in the treatment of a specific case and, of course, could give no good answer. Nearly penniless, friendless, Malpighi died in 1694 some century and a half before the proper retort could be given to his questioners.

Sydenham (1624-1689), the puritan Oxford graduate, revived bedside medicine in England. A friend of Robert Boyle the chemist and John Locke the philosopher, Sydenham was no friend of theories or respecter of authorities, except Hippocrates. The work of Vesalius, Harvey and Malpighi was unknown to him or ignored; his favorite authors besides Hippocrates were Bacon, Cicero and Cervantes, whose *Don Quixote* he recommended to a medical student who asked him which book he should read. His descriptions of scarlet fever (as named and distinguished by him from measles for the first time), of rheumatic chorea, and of his own gout are classic. Sydenham advocated fresh air in sickrooms, a treatment then unknown, and recommended iron therapy for chlorosis, the then prevalent anemia of young women.

The eighteenth century saw many advances in the identification of diseases and in techniques. Auenbrugger (1722-1809) published his book on percussion in 1761, adding another method of physical examination to the inspection and auscultation of ancient times. Thermometry began to be applied clinically to a greater degree and the "fever" of ancient ages began to be studied more carefully. Surgery, largely in the hands of the barbers, rose slowly as a discipline, and as late as 1744 Frederick the Great of Prussia confirmed the right of the Prussian executioner to set fractures and heal wounds. In John Hunter (1728-1793) scientific study of diseases began to be associated with surgery and experimental surgery was founded by this nearly universal genius whose contributions to comparative anatomy and experimental pathology are only two of a great variety that can be mentioned. Linnaeus (1707-1778) applied his methods of classification to plants, to animals and finally to diseases, not the first in this regard by any means but the first who used classification as an end in itself.

No country in Europe was lacking distinguished clinical practitioners of great capabilities. England had more than her share, but besides Pringle a pupil of Boerhaave, the founder of military medicine and of the Red Cross; Withering of the foxglove (digitalis) for dropsy; Jenner of smallpox fame and many others, the name and fame of William Heberden (1710-1801) stand out. Dr. Johnson of the dictionary was asked on his deathbed "who was his physician?" and answered, "Heberden of course, *ultimus Romanorum*—the last of the Romans." His recognition and description of angina pectoris (1768) is classic but he is remembered also by the nodes he described on the fingers in rheumatism. In France, Jean Nicholas Corvisart (1755-1821) began the application of autopsy correlations with clinical observations, to be continued so successfully by the shortlived genius René Laennec (1786-1821) who was to introduce the stethoscope as an aid in auscultation as well as to describe the liver disease since bearing his name, "Laennec's Cirrhosis."

As described previously, the publication of Morgagni's autopsy series in 1761 and of Baillie's systematic organ pathology in 1793 began the development of modern pathology. Medicine began the study of the changes underlying and producing the signs and symptoms of disease which was to culminate in 1858 in the cellular pathology of Rudolf Virchow. If this were a history of men rather than of ideas one could not neglect such great physicians as Bright, Addison, Graves, Hodgkin and Parry in the British Isles. Bouillaud, Ricord, Richet and Pinel in France could not be left out, nor Wunderlich (who found fever a disease and left it a symptom), Skoda, Hebra, Holmes, Semmelweis, Bigelow and Drake, and many others, nor could this chapter be kept to a reasonable size.

But in studying ideas one can not truly say that modern medicine differs in many essential regards from that of a century ago, except in one area to be discussed a little later. Radiology has been added to our methods for the study of patients, as have the aids of the clinical pathology laboratory in bacteriology, hematology, clinical chemistry, surgical pathology and the study of biopsies and smears. Some combinations are being made as chemistry teams up with histology in histochemistry. The refinements of the laboratory—automation, tagging by radioisotopes and the search for the ever smaller with the electron microscopes—are added to the investigation of disease.

But our viewpoints in the consideration of disease have not changed a great deal in any essential feature except one, the return of the *psyche* as a subject of study. The pioneer studies of mental disease by Charcot, by Kraepelin and by Weir Mitchell in the last century and by Freud, Jung, Adler and Adolph Meyer among many others in this one, have added a new, more than a little speculative, dimension to the clinical considerations of physicians. Psychosomatic diseases and the psychic "overlays" or "underlays" of many organic diseases are being appreciated more and more. The actual sad fact is that in our study of the diseases and disorders of the mind we have relatively little objective data for the good reason that characteristic cellular or chemical changes have not yet been elucidated for the majority of mental disturbances. Until this happy eventuality is reached, psychiatry is going along as clinical medicine went along for centuries, with workable theories but without complete success. The emergence of the current group of psychiatrists equally acquainted with the laboratory bench and with the analyst's couch gives promise of better days to come.

There is current active interest in the classification of disease, impelled in large part by the demands of governmental agencies and life insurance companies which require large amounts of easily recoverable data for their efficient operation. Another impetus to classification is in the potential use of computer-type machines for the processing of data covering the frequency of disease and even for the diagnosis of disease itself. This goes along with the current stirrings among the taxonomic biologists and among the microbiologists, who are beginning to use the computers in many problems.

The microbiologists have returned to a system of classification first proposed in 1763 by the French botanist, Michel Adanson, for plants. In this scheme all possible data are utilized: size, shape, staining ability, genetic constitution, growth requirements, fermentation reactions, and so on, almost *ad infinitum*, sometimes with two hundred descriptors and with a *minimum* of forty or fifty. This is reviewed in the XIIth symposium of the Society of General Microbiology (1962) by P.H.A. Sneath. One result of such an analysis, of interest to pathologists, is the combination of Nocardia and Mycobacterium into one large group.

In clinical medicine we discuss today as disease entities a great number of conditions named in the past, sometimes long ago, before modern laboratory and other aids were available. These "platonic figures," these ideas we call diseases, may have alternative taxonomies which the sorting of data by some mechanical aid, such as computers, could reveal. Some tumors have aspects of infections, for example. The entities classed as the so-called collagen diseases have a heterogeneous complexity that represents either over-classification or under-discrimination. Perhaps the present classification of diseases, based on such diverse headings in the International Nomenclature as etiology, anatomy or just local custom, will in time be replaced by some more logical grouping derived from the computer.

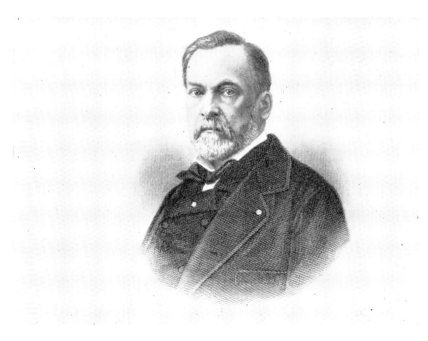

Pasteur (1822-1895)—Father of Bacteriology.

Chapter 7

Certain Diseases Are Known to Have Specific Etiologies and All Diseases Are Caused

HE BELIEF that certain diseases have specific etiologies is quite ancient, and upon it, therapy is based rationally. In earliest history, as among our contemporary or recent primitive people, the causes of disease are believed to be hostile magic, evil spirit or demonic possession. Among the Ancient Egyptians it is recorded in a medical papyrus that a physician told the patient, "Death has entered your body." The Winnebago Indians, a branch of the Sioux tribes, has a legend of "Deathgiver," the greatest of Gods. Whereas the Assyrian legends told of a time at which there was no death or disease, in the 2nd millenium disease was known and was already blamed on the all-powerful gods who allow diseases to happen. The idea of disease as an affliction for a sin or transgression is present in the older books of the Hebrew Bible.

Poisons appear to be among the materials first recognized in antiquity to cause disease and death. The word used in Homer, *pharmakon*, refers to a drug which is healing or noxious. In the Odyssey it is said, "... the fertile soil of Egypt is most rich in drugs, many of which are wholesome in fashion, although many are poisons." In the Hippocratic corpus and thereafter, physicians in Greece recognized poisons of natural origin and the venoms of animals as capable of causing disease and death, as well as a variety of other causes less definite in our eyes, meteorologic, climatic and geographic conditions. Theophrastus, Aristotle's pupil, knew that an extract of mistletoe was poisonous while hemlock had been used to kill Socrates. Hemlock was also used as a narcotic, as were opium and a number of other materials. Nicander, a Greek of the 2nd century B.C., wrote a poem "Alexipharmaca" dealing with poisons and their antidotes. In Imperial Rome professional poisoners flourished, as described by Livy and by Cicero, while the Jewish sage, Moses Maimonides, wrote a book on poisons in 1199. A little later in the west, Peter of Abano (1250-1316) wrote *de Venenis*, on poisons, which included a wide variety of those already mentioned, but also both menstrual and leprous blood. Professional poisoners were rampant in France and Italy in the 16th and 17th centuries and it was during this period that the Florentine Borgias acquired the dubious distinction of being the world's worst hosts until superseded by the Campbells in relation to the MacDonalds in the Glencoe episode.

Not much more concerning poisons as causes of disease was added until relatively recent times, although from a different viewpoint Vitruvius, the architect of Rome, had spoken of a disease of lead workers. The final step in the inculpation of lead as a poison was accomplished by Baker in 1767 in the Devonshire colic endemic among those drinking cider which had been contaminated with lead from the apple presses during its manufacture. Agricola (1490-1555) in his *de Metallica* spoke of the illnesses peculiar to miners. Claude Bernard in 1853-58 wrote of carbon monoxide poisoning with the gas displacing oxygen from the erythrocytes, and Wormley wrote of the microchemistry of poisons in 1867. By this time an industrial toxicology was beginning; this was most prominent in the first half of the nineteenth century, and it has continued to implicate a variety of materials used in industry as causes of diseases ranging from silica, bauxite fumes, cotton and sugar cane fibers, and many dusts, to chemicals such as carbon tetrachloride and naphthylamine. The list of noxious chemicals has been enlarged recently by the addition of insecticides and pesticides in great variety and number, many of which have been shown to be capable of poisoning people.

The story of the discovery of the role of living organisms as specific causes of disease is an interesting one, foreshadowed by theories and confusion. Individuals with disease called "leprosy" have been separated and isolated from the general population since Assyrian and Biblical times. This process continued during the middle ages and into relatively recent times. This precaution is now taken with cases of Hansen's disease, the current leprosy. The plagues and epidemics were suspected of being transmitted by some way from person to person during the centuries until the 16th. There are intimations of an understanding of the ways in which this was accomplished, notably by two Moors (one of Almeria and the other of Granada), while da Foligro in Italy spoke of germs of disease in the Black Death epidemics. Quarantine, isolating a traveler to Marseilles for forty days, was instituted in 1383 to prevent the introduction of disease.

Girolamo Fracastoro (1483-1553), described by Bullock as "a scholar, a poet and a thinker," began the serious study of contagion in his book of the same name, a little quarto volume containing only 77 pages, published in 1546. This gentleman of Verona is perhaps beter known for his poem (1530) "*Syphilis sive Morbus Gallicus*" in which he describes the afflicted shepherd and gave a name to the new disease which had appeared in Spain following the completion of Columbus' second voyage and then was carried to Sicily and Italy by Spanish troops and their entourage. In his book on contagion, Fracastoro not only recognized the role of direct contact in the transmission of disease but introduced the word *Fomites* (from *fomes*, touchstone or tinder) for the clothing, dishes and utensils which had been used by the patient and which could transmit the disease. In an early reference to renascent atomism, Fracastoro spoke of "atoms" of infection but other important observations are included, for example that individuals are usually only once attacked by variola and measles,—". . . it is rare for people who have had these diseases to have them again."

Pasteur in the later third of the 19th century showed that bacteria could cause disease, a far step from the theory of Fracastoro but one which proceeded in an interesting fashion, demonstrating the convergence of several lines of thought. Kircher (1601-1680), a German Jesuit, spoke of an effluvium of small, imperceptible, living bodies, while his friend Lange (1619-1662) introduced the idea of *pathologia animatum*, that disease could be caused by the entry into an individual of small living bodies. Leeuwenhoek (1632-1723) probably saw bacteria with his primitive microscope in 1674, but these *animalicules* were not to be associated with disease for two centuries. The Abbé de Sault in the 1740's had said that tuberculosis was caused by small worms, and was only infectious in the later stages when those small agents were numerous.

Spontaneous generation—the origin of living forms from inanimate matter—was still held as a matter of belief until the experiments of Pasteur (1822-1895) in 1861, but originated with Aristotle or before him. It had first to be shown by Schwann in 1836 that putrefaction was caused by living agents and that yeast, used in fermentation, was also alive, again accomplished by Schwann, as well as by deTour in 1837. Ehrenburg nearly a century before had studied microorganisms of the sort which the Italian Bassi (1773-1856) had shown to cause a disease in silkworms in 1836. By 1840, Jacob Henle (1809-1885), best known as the discoverer of the tubule loops in the kidney named after him, could build up a contagious-infectious theory of disease implicating microorganisms. There was the resistance of centuries of thought to overcome. Even an early experiment by Rayer who inoculated an ass with pus from a patient with glanders (1838), the animal dying in nine days, did not convince the skeptics, notable among whom were the physiologists led by Magendie in Paris. It required the painstaking techniques of Cohn and Koch and the isolation, staining and culturing of the organisms before they could be proven to cause disease. Experimental replicas of human disease had to be produced by using bacteria in experimental animals, studied and sectioned for microscopic study, with recovery of the organisms in culture.

Other living agents, ranging from the viruses (shown in 1892 to cause the mosaic disease of tobacco plants, and in 1897, the foot-and-mouth disease of cattle and requiring living cells for their growth) to fungi, rickettsia, protozoa and many other forms have since been studied in human disease. Viruses can now be examined with the immense magnifying power of the electron microscope while similar agents infecting bacteria, bacteriophages, have been discovered and are being studied by every means available.

I have omitted telling of many of the false steps in the development of bacteriology and it would not do to recount many of the incorrect surmises which have followed the discovery that bacteria and other living agents can cause disease. As a warning against too readily implicating any living agent as a *cause*, merely because it has been found *in* a lesion, we need to recall the suggestions that Brucella caused Hodgkin's disease, that *Mycobacterium tuberculosis* caused rheumatoid arthritis and a great number of other diseases, and that the Streptococcus caused a variety of diseases ranging from poliomyelitis to rheumatoid arthritis to ulcerative colitis and so on almost *ad infinitum*. Charles Darwin said that, "Nature will delude one at every possible opportunity;" this seems to happen most frequently when the relationships of living organisms to each other are being studied.

That immunity could be acquired against a disease was established by William Jenner (1749-1823) who after 1796 used inoculation with cowpox to protect against smallpox. The tale is told that a dairy maid had imparted to Jenner the countryfolk's knowledge that an attack of cowpox protected one against smallpox and that John Hunter had inspired to actual testing. Earlier, the diarist Lady Wortley Montagu had introduced into England vaccination with dried smallpox pus which she had observed in use in Turkey where her husband was the British ambassador. Because of an occasional death resulting from this method of vaccination, the practice never became popular. In 1880 Pasteur observed that an old culture of cholera organisms did not produce the usual and characteristic disease when injected into fowl, and further that the animals which were so treated did not develop the disease when injected with fresh virulent organisms. Immunity had been developed by the accidental "attenuation" of the bacteria, and the principle was established that organisms could be altered so that on injection they would not produce the disease but would rather induce the animal to develop protection against them. Following this observation, quite a number of bacterial diseases were controlled; diphtheria, typhoid fever, tetanus and cholera were among the many. More recently, virus diseases are beginning to submit to such treatment; the poliomyelitis viruses, treated by heat in the Salk method or attenuated by culture under unfavorable circumstances in the Sabin method, are being used for mass immunizations which promise to wipe out this once formidable scourge.

Not all blessings are unmixed and by 1902 Richet in France and Theobald Smith in the United States had demonstrated that injections of some materials into animals do not induce the expected protective immunity but rather increase the susceptibility of the animal to it. This reaction termed Allergy by Richet, to describe an altered reaction, has since been implicated in the causation of a number of important human diseases ranging from asthma and hay-fever to a great number of both skin and visceral diseases.

It is now clear that the induction of an immune state is caused by, or accompanied by the appearance of, a particular and specific type of protein in the blood of the immunized animal, human or otherwise. This new protein is closely related to, but not identical with, one normally present in the serum of the animal. The stimuli to the production of the antibody or new protein is the antigen of injected protein; the study of the factors concerned is called Immunology. It has been realized that Immunology plays a role in such diverse procedures as blood transfusions and attempts at tissue and organ transplantation between individuals. A whole area of study has been opened, notably by the Nobel Prize winners, Sir Mac-Farlane Burnet and P. B. Medawar who investigated the Self and Non-Self relationship, as Burnet calls it, the problem of individuality or separate identity by which an organism "recognizes" that an injected protein is, or is not, identical with its own proteins.

It is remarkable, in a way, that an understanding of disease caused by a deficient intake of necessary foods—i.e., nutritional disease—is of recent attainment, mostly accomplished in this century. The views of the Egyptians on the role of foods in causing diseases as described by Herodotus, has already been mentioned. The Assyrians are quoted by Sigerist as saying: "Fasting, abstinence from food and drink afflict the mind; illness follows." Nutrition assumed major importance for the Greeks and special treatises on diet appear for the first time. In the collection of works of the Hippocratic school of physicians, the Hippocratic Corpus as it is called, dating back to the 5th century B.C., starvation is listed as one of the causes of disease. Further, Aristotle's views on the soul as forming the basis for life are basic in the philosopher's ideas, and the fundamental soul is the nutritive or vegetative soul on which growth depends. Only this nutritive soul is possessed by vegetables and plants while animals have in addition a "sensitive" or sensible soul and the human being has as well a "rational" soul with powers of abstraction and reflection. The views of Aristotle may be summarized as follows:

Vegetables—Nutritive or Vegetative soul—Growth.

Animals—Nutritive soul and Sensitive soul—Growth and Movement.

Human Beings—Nutritive soul, Sensitive soul, Rational soul—Growth, Movement, and Thought.

The Hippocratic Corpus emphasized diet in the treatment of disease states. Hippocrates said "Undernourishment gives rise to many troubles and, though they are different from those produced by over-eating, they are nonetheless severe because they are more diverse and more specific." The influence, as transmitted in the writings of the Alexandrian physicians and of Galen, Celsus, and Orobasius, prevailed until the Scientific Revolution of the 15th, 16th, 17th and 18th centuries, and beyond. Mass episodes of starvation occurred throughout the time intervening from Ancient Greece to nearly modern Europe, associated with unfavorable climatic conditions and ineffectual distributive methods for foods in many instances. All too often man-made famines followed the ravages of war or occurred in besieged cities, starvation being used as a weapon to force surrender.

It is rare to find any mention in medical writings to the effect that deficiency apart from complete starvation can cause disease, despite the fact that many diseases we recognize as being nutritional are to be found in them. Scurvy, caused by deficiency of ascorbic acid or vitamin C, can be recognized frequently, especially in the accounts of the voyages of exploration after the discovery of America. Chlorosis, an anemia of young women caused by iron deficiency, can be recognized readily while the goiters or neck swelling of the Alpine inhabitants resulting from Iodine deficiency have been known and remarked upon since Roman times: "Quis guttitur in Alpis?" Actually, in ancient times it was known that ground-up sponges and dried and pulverized seaweed, both good sources of iodine, were good therapeutic agents for the goiters but the role of iodine or even the existence of such an element was not known. Sydenham recommended iron for the anemia of chlorosis, for a reason not known, while Trousseau (1801-1867), using iron for the same condition, thought of it as a "tonic" rather than as a specific substance satisfying a deficiency.

The first vitamin effect recorded is that scurvy could be prevented by the addition of lime or lemon to the diet, as demonstrated by the British naval surgeon, Lind (1716-1794), in 1757. The disease appeared in epidemics among troops in barracks or sailors on long voyages during the days of sail. It was nearly forty years after the discovery and recommendation of Lind before the Admiralty added the preventive citrus fruits to the sailors' rations. It is interesting that Jacques Cartier's band of French explorers in Canada, afflicted with scurvy in the winter of 1535, inquired of the Indians for a remedy and were successfully treated with some uncertain vegetable extract, possibly made from spruce needles.

The term vitamin (originally spelled with a terminal "e") was introduced by Funk to describe a factor absent in polished rice but present in the native rice, the deficiency of which caused the disease beriberi, prevalent in the Orient where rice is a dietary staple and protein is in short supply. The suggestion was made by Funk that not only was scurvy also a disease caused by vitamin deficiency, but that pellagra and rickets were as well. Pellagra known as *Mal de la Rose* and other names was a disease that appeared with the introduction of maize or Indian corn from the New World into European diets after Columbus' voyages, in Egypt in the 1840's when the corn reached that country, and in the U.S.A. in the 1800's. A considerable amount of study was required before Goldberger showed after 1926 that the severe disease, characterized by the three D's—dermatitis, diarrhea and dementia—was the result of a deficiency of niacin or nicotinic acid. The role of corn in producing pellagra is still obscure and there is a strong possibility of an anti-nicotinic acid, a pellagrogenic factor, being present in it. Rickets has been known for centuries and it has been suggested that its name comes from the Anglo-Saxon word meaning "to twist," referring to the bent and bowed legs of the affected child. Dellarobia's infants, tightly wrapped to prevent distortion, are a witness to the prevalence in Renaissance Italy of the disease, now known to result from a deficiency of Vitamin D and preventable by a supply of cod liver oil.

A multitude of other vitamins and their part in the genesis and treatment of human disease have been discovered, so many in fact that the list is too long to be included here. Additionally, metal deficiencies in the diet are beginning to be recognized in addition to those of iron and iodine already described. Further, amino acid and protein-deficiency states in man are being hypothesized and the evidence for their existence is increasingly good. It is rather distressing to discover that the laboratory rat can choose a balanced diet from materials supplied to him and that the primitive Bantu, before the arrival of civilization, was able to keep in nutritional balance, but that the contemporary Bantu, like his brothers of the older civilization, is unable to keep his diet adequate.

Of considerable interest in nutrition is the recognition of nutritional deficit in the convalescent patient after a severe illness or following major surgery. It is not hyperbole to point out that such individuals are living off their body proteins just as much as starving persons in a famine-ravaged country or the prisoners of the concentration camps of World War II. The necessity of the restoration to nutritional balance of these convalescent patients, who are literally "starving in the midst of plenty," has assumed considerable importance in current surgery and represents a recent accomplishment of nutritional study.

The Evolutionary Theory of Charles Darwin (1809-1882), introduced like Virchow's Cell Theory in the eventful year of 1858, could not fail to influence thinking in the medical sciences. The mutability of species had been suggested by individuals ranging from St. Augustine, Goethe, Oken, von Baer and Lamarck to Lyell, Chambers and Spencer. The possible influence of heredity on the occurrence of disease had been long considered, especially since breeding methods had been used for thousands of years for deliberate selections of desirable characteristics in domestic animals. The Chinese had been breeding garden flowers, most notably the rose, for a thousand years, and Columbus described the Indians' selection of their desirable forms of maize. In the 18th century new emphasis and efforts were devoted in England and in Europe on breeding of animals and plants.

The Austrian monk, Gregor Mendel (1822-1884), experimented between 1857 to 1868 on the crossing of sweet peas, and selected certain simple qualities for study, the tallness or shortness of the plants. In publications between 1866 and 1869 he stated a series of laws of heredity but these discoveries received little notice until rediscovered by DeVries in 1902. It is customary to explain the neglect of Mendel's epoch-making discoveries on their publication in obscure journals but such is not in fact the case. Not only were some of the papers published in widely read journals but reprints are said to have been sent to distinguished biologists. The more likely truth is that the time was not ripe for the acceptance of Mendel's laws; this is suggested further by the finding of the pages uncut in the journal number bearing one of Mendel's articles in the library of one of the world's great universities.

Whatever the cause for the long neglect of Mendel's studies, after 1900 research in genetics, the science of heredity, flourished and became increasingly productive. The chromosomes occurring during cell division were recognized in 1888, and discovered by Van Beneden to have a constant number in each species, the number for different species ranging from a very few to several hundred. The studies of T. H. Morgan, Bateson, Johannsen and Castle further elaborated Mendel's laws and began the process of relating the hypothetic carriers of Mendel's factors, the genes, to the chromosomes of Flemming. Progress is rapid in this field in human disease at the present time, E. B. Ford and others having shown the association of genetic anomaly with human disease.

The "Inborn Errors of Metabolism"—alkaptonuria, cystinuria, pentosuria and albinism—described by Garrod in 1908, have since been demonstrated to be genetically determined and to these four a great many more have been added, ranging from the metabolic disturbance of uric acid in gout to Sickle Cell disease. The problem raised by such a discovery has both moral and ethical as well as medical implications, yielding yet another riddle for the human race to solve. Added to this demonstration of the influence of breeding on the appearance of human disease has been the suggested probability that some disturbances of the heart and other viscera can result from maternal disease during pregnancy. The "benign" exanthem, German measles, has been implicated, especially when it occurs during a crucial few weeks early in pregnancy. What we now have to face is that the fetus during certain stages of development will have the same diseases that the mother has. Further, at least one drug has been found to produce serious distortions and deficiencies in the limb development of the fetus when taken by the mother early in pregnancy. Undoubtedly other similar causes, and most likely among them maternal nutritional deficiency, will be found in time.

Diseases in some instances, as in the drug-produced limb disturbances in the fetus, may be iatrogenic or physician-induced by the therapy. The dangers of the pyramidon drugs, of the sulfonamides, penicillin and many other antibiotics, of blood transfusions, or virus transmission by needles causing hepatitis, have induced much concern in the minds of many physicians. A concerted effort is presently being made to minimize the frequency of such unfortunate accidents, the efforts being based most realistically on a constant awareness of such dangers.

The development of psychosomatic medicine and the introduction of Selye's concept of stress in the production of disease have combined to raise the possibility that factors which at present we can only call psychologic may be important in medical etiology. John Hunter's prediction, "My life is at the mercy of any fool who chooses to make me angry," later fulfilled, is familiar to most physicians as exemplifying the influence of emotion on heart disease. To heart disease we now must add asthma, many varieties of skin diseases, various types of peptic ulceration, and a number of other conditions whose psychosomatic basis is now more than suggested.

We can boast that we do know the cause of a growing number of diseases—trauma, poisons, living agents, immunity, dietary deficiencies, genetic defects and developmental influences, as well as psychic influences. At the same time we must state fairly that the cause of human cancer is quite unknown except in the case of a relatively few varieties, and that the causes of many important and prevalent types of diseases of the heart and blood vessels quite escape our comprehension at present. Further, much remains to be learned about the ways in which obvious causes of disease produce their effects. "Much has been done by those who went before, but much still remains to be done," as Seneca says, so that the opportunities for the search and attainment of new knowledge in medicine should not be wanting within the span of human existence on this planet.

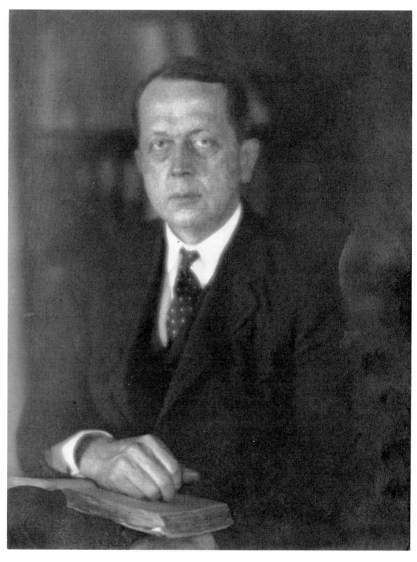

MacCallum (1874-1944)—Disease in the Whole Body.

(From the Author's Collection.)

Chapter 8

Appropriate Treatment Can Benefit the Individual Patient and in Many Cases Cure the Disease

HE AIM of Medicine has always been the relief of the sick person. This objective implies the belief that it is possible to accomplish such amelioration, and statements to this effect can be found from Hippocrates to Harrison. The sage of Cos says:

> "I would define (the aims of) Medicine as the complete removal of the distress of the sick, the alleviation of the more violent diseases and the refusal to undertake to cure cases in which the disease has already won the mastery."

Harrison and his co-authors in their introductory chapter have this to say:

> "The practicing physician must never forget that his primary and traditional objectives are utilitarian—the prevention and cure of disease and the relief of suffering, whether of body or mind."

Apart from a rather more optimistic viewpoint, the inclusion of the preventive aspect, and the realization that some suffering is mental as opposed to physical (a distinction that the Greeks did not make), the aims of the Harrison group agree with the Hippocratic corpus. In general the same thought is stated by Florey:

> "The main reason why a patient sees a doctor is to be relieved of his symptoms. His medical attendant endeavors to do this by

therapeutic procedures which may be directed to relieving the symptoms or, more rationally, to dealing with the underlying cause."

The statement by Florey of the doctor's task is not much different than that of either Hippocrates or Harrison's group, with the addition of the pathologist's belief that it is important to separate the relief of symptoms from the treatment of the basic disease. The history of the fundamental ideas in medicine can be traced in these three statements as they represent the purposes or ends of medicine—the treatment and cure of disease and of the patient.

It will be appreciated readily that rational therapy of the ill individual depends on a reasonable identification and understanding both of the person and of his disease. For many centuries there was lacking the proper understanding of the nature and features of disease as has already been pointed out; disease was regarded as the effect of a demoniac possession, as caused by a maldistribution of body fluids or humors; speculation was proportional to the lack of exact knowledge. In these circumstances there was a dearth of rational treatment and one might suppose that, little information being available, care of the sick was inadequate and inefficient. As will be shown, this was not the case. The ability of the body to recover by itself from disease has been forgotten. One needs only to search the medical journals, say of the eighteenth century, to appreciate what capacities for healing are possessed by the human being. Further, a great deal was done for patients, many disease processes were identified and relatively specific therapy for different disease states appeared from time to time. Finally, the audacity of the surgeon has not been a recent development; despite lack of adequate anaesthesia or of understanding of infection or of blood or fluid replacement, for three thousand years or more individuals have had the temerity to attempt to remove almost any diseased organ or to drain suppuration wherever placed, stimulated by the belief that such heroic measures (especially heroic as far as the patient was concerned) might affect a cure.

It has been said that few operations were performed in 1900 that were not done in Graeco-Roman antiquity. There is an element of hyperbole in this statement which might have been made by a physician, but again operations were done in Graeco-Roman times that would not have been done in 1900. The Hippocratic corpus tells us of the handling of fractures and dislocations and splinting, and in ancient Greece thoracentesis, paracentesis and operations on fistula and on hemorrhoids were performed. The cutting for the stone, i.e., removal of vesical calculi, was forbidden by the Hippocratic code, being left to the ordinary practitioners of the operation, apparently another group. Surgery in Rome included amputations using a flap, ligature of vessels, herniotomies, umbilical and inguinal hernias in children, craniotomies for epilepsy and for possible hemorrhage or suppuration, in fact an almost endless list. There are even descriptions of hysterectomies and pneumonectomies while mammectomies for cancer (or scirrhus) of the breast date back to Greece. The Ebers papyrus of 1550 B.C. contains a description, apparently of a thyroidectomy, performed by an Egyptian specialist. John Hunter described (1781) tube-feeding as an innovation; actually it had been known in Graeco-Roman medicine, and Fabricius ab Aquapendente (1537-1619) had described and illustrated the use of a nasal tube for the purpose.

Therapy in surgery remained speculative, and based on what now seems to be irrational speculation, but some elements of good sense were present. Cauterization of dog bites had been done since antiquity, reasonably enough in view of the danger of rabies, but cauterization of all gunshot wounds, on the basis that they were all "poisoned," seems less reasonable. The advance in thought represented by the decision of Ambrose Paré (1510-1590), the great French surgeon, to do away with cauterization or irrigation of the wound with boiling oil, after observing that the lack of the oil treatment made the wound heal better, would have been thought a considerable advance in treatment and thinking, if he had not subsequently treated the wound with Dioscorides' (1st century) earthworm ointment, different only in that puppy fat was substituted for goose grease. He is reported to have treated burns with onions. Even including that sort of treatment, Paré's skill was a high point in the history of surgery until relatively recent times.

Osler said about 1900 that "From Hippocrates to Hunter, the treatment of disease was one long traffic in hypotheses." Doctrines of sympathy and antipathy or contrasts prevailed for centuries; the custom of treating the weapon with medicine while the wound which it caused was being similarly treated was long in favor. Astrology was held to give useful information about the patient for many centuries; the positions of the moon, stars and sun at the time of the patient's birth and during his illness influenced the type and amount of therapy. Polypharmacy, the compounding of the prescriptions containing many drugs, was in practice into the present centuries. Within the last few centuries such materials as dried and powdered blood, moss, ground-up human skulls, the treacle compound *mithridatium*, and *bezoar*, the calculus found in the stomach of some animals, disappeared pretty well from the pharmacopeia of most reputable physicians.

Bleeding from a vein was in use from the time of Hippocrates until the last century. A leading and most popular textbook of medicine about 1840 said:

> "Of all the treatments in medicine, the most efficacious is the letting of blood; stand the patient upright and bleed from the ante-cubital vein until syncope occurs."

Among the famous who were sped to their fathers by the practice of bleeding was George Washington, severely ill with a throat infection that sounds like diphtheria. Blood letting was probably useful in some cases of hypertension and in polycythemia while not positively harmful in any number of trivial illnesses. It is unlikely that blood letting was of any great help in any sizeable proportion of the innumerable cases in which it was practiced over the span of two thousand years and more.

The autopsies of Morgagni and the systematized pathology of Baillie, both in the period of John Hunter, deserve credit as the beginning of scientific medicine. The data from other biologic sciences and the way of thinking which followed the scientific revolution of the sixteenth century gave bases for the viewpoint of Virchow and for the discoveries of the founders of modern chemistry, microbiology, physiology and anatomy. "The traffic in hypotheses" of which Osler spoke really ended with the rise of scientific medicine, practically within the last hundred years. The medical application of the scientific viewpoint still continues and is not yet complete.

Up to this point in our discussion of treatment in the present chapter we have emphasized the shortcomings of our medical ancestors. We have described the scope and diversity of the therapeutic materials and attempts, and the wrong, when not obviously inane, hypotheses on which treatment was based. We have mentioned audacity in the centuries of surgical attempts, by surgeons proper and barber-surgeons and just plain charlatans, who waged mighty attacks on the suffering human body without adequate anaesthesia, antisepsis or asepsis and without having knowledge of physiology but with an unbounded confidence surpassing even that of their complacent medical contemporaries.

Yet solid accomplishments were made in the medical sciences in the millenia up to the rise of scientific medicine in the 19th century, and it is important for us to realize this. Some of this information came from misguided attempts at therapy, "now hitting the disease and now the patient," as Osler says; and the close attendance to, and study of, the patient with the limited means available produced a harvest of information on which we still in large part depend.

The identification and recognition of disease patterns for many of the common diseases came into the armamentarium of medicine in the period during which measures to modify the course of disease were yet unavailable. A great many of the phenomena in the contest between the disease process and the human body were recognized, described and discussed so that they became a part of the basic learning required of the medical student, such as fever, prognostic signs, and relations between apparently disparate symptoms. As Snapper eloquently says, there is in the precipitous onrush of scientific medicine a real danger that some of this information may be disregarded and lost. To put it another way, we may forget all of our gains about the natural history of disease in the patient while we learn more about the scientific aspects of disease.

Before the rise of truly scientific medicine, the beginning of anatomy, following the pioneer works of Vesalius, Fallopius and Harvey, gave a structural basis on which many facts of disease could be considered. Important features in gross anatomy were discovered and in time they were associated with fundamental physiologic observations so that an image of the "machine man" was formed in the physician's mind. The later addition of chemistry and of more details of the finer structure of the body added to and built upon the fundamental discoveries of several centuries. Further, the explanation of disease in a number of instances on an anatomic-physiologic basis is still possible, following the pattern set by our predecessors.

Various therapeutic procedures, including the use of a limited number of efficacious drugs and of a great number of surgical interventions, were shown to be feasible in the sick person. Many of the drugs, such as digitalis, opium and various mineral derivatives, still play a considerable role in therapy. The scientific investigation of the modes of action of these materials and their effects on the living human and other animals and on isolated portions of them have served to establish laboratory methods of great precision and have produced solid information. The surgery of the past, as well as demonstrating the endurance of the human being and his resistance to trauma, was useful in that a great many if not all of the current surgical procedures were tried out on human beings. Today a surgeon in training or in developing a new operation will test it on an animal in the laboratory and will then apply it to the human being when the kinks have been worked out and the *modus operandi* seems not to injure the animal. The early surgeons with very few exceptions, and many of these in antiquity, applied the operation to the patient when once they had conceived of the way in which it could be done.

In a very real sense, then, the early history of medicine and that up until the relatively recent development of its scientific aspects can be thought of as a period of laboratory experimentation in which were discovered the broader features of the human patient, what could be done for him, and what the body could tolerate. This was not all, for the major patterns of the medical disciplines were set up, the special areas in which concentrated study and practice were required—Medicine, Surgery, Obstetrics, Gynecology, Pediatrics, Ophthalmology, and Otolaryngology, as well as Orthopedic Surgery and the rest of the clinical specialties as well as the basic science disciplines of Anatomy, Physiology, Biochemistry, Pathology, Microbiology, Pharmacology, and so on. These were not set up by a committee either of government or of a medical association but they grew up in the most reasonable fashion possible; they developed in response to needs.

Modern medicine has admittedly made great strides in the prevention and treatment of disease. In surgery, the operator has the advantage of medical, microbiologic and physiologic controls and he has the guidance of the surgical pathologist, "backed-up" by the hospital tissue committee to prevent his lapsing into the exuberances of his predecessors. To help him in his patient care, during the operation his environment is kept as close to aseptic as possible, in keeping with the 1861 observation of Pasteur that bacteria cause putrefaction, probably the bacteria which Koch had found in 1878 in surgical sepsis. Superseding the attempted antisepsis of Joseph Lord Lister (1827-1912) with zinc chloride and then carbolic acid, the more reasonable asepsis produced by sterilization followed the introduction of steam sterilization by von Bergmann (1836-1907) in 1886. Röentgen's X-ray (1896) is in frequent use by the surgeon, many times with the image-amplifier to aid him. The return of the surgeon to scientific medicine has resulted in the elevation of his craft.

From the viewpoint of the surgical patient's well-being, the introduction of anaesthesia and an understanding of the special features of the period of recovery or convalescence after injury or operation are most important. General anaesthesia came into use as the result of the activities of the Hartford dentist, Horace Wells (1815-1848), who administered nitrous oxide for a tooth extraction in 1844 and of Crawford Long (1815-1878) of Georgia who in 1842 removed a neck tumor under ether anaesthesia. Chloroform was used by Simpson, the Edinburgh surgeon, about the same time. Local anesthesia was introduced by the great Hopkins surgeon, W. S. Halsted (1852-1922), in 1885 using cocaine, and spinal anaesthesia was first used by James Corning (1855-1923) and reported in the same year in the same volume (#42) of the same journal, the *New York State Journal of Medicine,* as was Halsted's contribution. The bodily phenomena which are consequent to a surgical operation of major severity or to a severe accident or a severe infection are much the same, as has been demonstrated recently. The changes in the circulation, and in the blood cells, and in the blood-clotting mechanisms have been known for twenty-five years or more but only in the last decade or so have the major metabolic disorders, involving the loss of body protein and a difficulty in restoring the loss, been appreciated—initially (1935) by the studies of Cuthbertson in England and more recently by Paul Cannon, Francis Moore and others in this country. There is probably some relationship to the secretions of the adrenal cortex during and after operation, injury or infection, which is perhaps related in turn to the stress condition described by Selye, but much remains to be done in this area. It is realized that the postoperative period is one of at least as much hazard to the patient as the operation itself, so that the day of the "operating-surgeon," the technician who saw the patient infrequently if at all after the operation, is rapidly and fortunately drawing to its close.

Internal Medicine has taken advantage of the advances in the scientific laboratories of the last century so that diseases are better diagnosed and more specifically treated than ever before. It is salutory to recall that Virchow who proposed the epoch-making cellular theory in 1858 said in 1847 that "since there are no specific disease entities, so there are no specific therapies." Quinine, specific against the malarial parasite, was already known and the last quarter of the 19th century found the appropriate antisera against diphtheria and tetanus. Particularly in the field of protective immunization has progress been great, culminating in the recent vaccines of Salk and Sabin, apparently preventing acute anterior poliomyelitis. Antibiotics of great variety, beginning with the synthesized sulfonamides and continuing with penicillin, and the "mycins" have poured from the laboratories into the physicians' hands and have speedily found their way into patients. That this therapy was not always needed, that it could be dangerous, and that new, resistant strains of organisms have developed following inadequate and inappropriate antibiotic therapy have been later and sobering conclusions of the medical team.

The emphasis on the treatment of the patient as a biologic unit is a development of great potential value, foreshadowed as it was by the emphasis on disease in the whole patient by the pathologist, W. G. MacCallum (1874-1944), and by Canby Robinson's *The Patient as a Person.* Such a viewpoint is in keeping with the modern biologist's conception of the Organism, as preached particularly by the so-called Organismic Biologists. Considered biologically, the upsurging Social Medicine is medical Ecology as indeed is Epidemiology, now being applied to the non-infectious diseases such as those of the heart and blood vessels and cancer, on a world-wide scale. The emphasis on the abnormalities of convalescence after surgery, trauma, and severe illness has a biologic aspect to it since the organism is presently viewed in the aspect of continuing development, the Developmental Biology of Paul Weiss and others, while earlier medical theory had considered the accident, the operation or the severe illness, as a complete episode.

Underlying and sparking the advances in Medicine and in Surgery has been a progressively accelerating addition of fundamental knowledge in the basic sciences, most notably in biochemistry, physiology and pathology. The idea of balance or stability or tendency to uniformity as characteristic of the living organism has been of great moment in modern medical thinking. The constancy of the internal environment of Claude Bernard and the Adaptation in Pathologic Processes of Welch had been synthesized into the Homeostasis of Walter B. Cannon and applied to the management of the ill and injured patient. Balance of salt and of water, and of nitrogen and most of the other measurable body chemicals, has become of great profitable utility in modern medical care, so that many lives have been saved as greater skill in the chemical manipulations has been attained. At the same time, as has been mentioned previously, the death of the patient "in perfect balance" is sufficiently frequent to remind the doctor that he is not dealing with a test tube but a human being. The role of the endocrine glands and the possibility of their supplementation when they are deficient in the patient, as well as a better understanding of their chemical structure, production and action are promised for the next period of medical advance.

The psychosomatic aspects of illness are presently being better appreciated than ever before by the great majority of doctors. The abnormality of the illness and the effect on the patient and on the social unit of which he is a part, as well as the even greater abnormality of the necessary hospital stay, are being recognized as considerably influencing the course and outcome of the illness.

Interestingly enough, the dictum to the experimentalists by the physicist, Nils Bohr, "The observation must not interfere with the thing observed," is being appreciated to apply to observations of the human organism quite as much as it does to the electron on which it is based. Medical students are being purposely introduced to the family as the proper social framework and home-care schemes are multiplying in use, not only because of shortage of hospital facilities but also because it is becoming more and more apparent that treatment of the patient in the home is less disruptive than institutional therapy, whenever this choice is possible.

One of the popular subjects of discussion in both medical and lay circles at the present time is the group of drugs, termed tranquillizers, intended to insulate the individual from the buffets of the world and the slings and arrows of outrageous fortune; in short, from stress. It is not likely that this ataraxic group of drugs was developed as a direct reaction to the theory of Selye, that stress of many sorts was an important and frequent cause of disease, but their popularization followed soon after his theory was first promulgated. Ataraxia, by the way, was the goal of the ancient Romans in the declining years of the empire: a state of being without cares and pleasantly indifferent to it all. The use of the tranquillizer group of drugs is so recent that only the rare severe injury, such as that of the liver with Thorazine®, has been recognized. The long-term effects of diminishing the sensitivity of the human being to the environmental stimuli on which his survival has hitherto depended, or more broadly, impeding one type of exchange between the organism and his environment which has until the present time been customary, cannot be predicted by me. The earlier tranquillizing drugs—alcohol, opium, and so on—have not been without harm to the individual and it is highly unlikely that psychiatrists will not become acquainted in time with conditions of disturbance resulting from the prolonged use of this frequently useful group of drugs.

I am least qualified to discuss the current status of psychiatry since the discipline has still a large element of non-objectivity to it; its data are appreciable only by one or a few individuals at a time and there have been to date no consistent tissue or cellular or body fluid change found in the most numerous of mental diseases.

The hallucinogenic drugs and the developing disciplines of psycho-pharmacology and psychochemistry give promise of an objective scientific investigation and explanation of mental disease which have been lacking up to the present time.

*A wound with a hot iron penetrating the pelvis;
by Dr.* ANDREW WILLISON, *phyſician at
Dundee.* Vol. IV. art. 15.

THE following hiſtory I chuſe to inſert, not as
it contains any new method of cure, but as it
ſhews that nature, but a little aſſiſted, cured a diſeaſe
which I looked on as deſperate. A ſmith, with a red-
hot iron in his hand, ran againſt a young fellow with
ſuch force, that it paſſed into the buttock an inch
and half from the anus, and came out through the
linea alba, an inch above the os pubis. When I
came to him, which was ſoon after the accident, I
found him with a low intermitting pulſe, bilious vomiting, pains in the belly, thirſt, cold ſweats, &c.
I ordered him to be blooded in a large quantity, and
a clyſter with turpentine to be thrown up, which gave
him ſome relief ; the next morning the ſymptoms
continued. I found he had made no urine, though he
had drank plentifully. His pulſe was quick and hard,
therefore I ordered him to be blooded again, and his
belly to be embrocated with oil of ſcorpions. Thirty
hours after he was wounded, he voided ſome urine re-
ſembling ſuch as people troubled with the ſtone do:
at night the clyſter was repeated, which brought away
a good deal of ſlime. He drank an emulſion with
nitre and a cordial julep, which check'd the violence
of the vomiting. The third day he uſed the embro-
cation, clyſter, &c. The urine and excrements now
came through the wound near the anus, into which I
injected a digeſting medicine with honey of roſes. In
ten days time the urine found its way through the
penis ; in ten days more the excrements came through
the anus, and in ſix weeks he was perfectly well.

A case report of 1747. Before scientific medicine.

(From the Author's collection.)

Chapter 9

Summary and Conclusions—Past, Present and Future

N THIS book we have presented the history of a series of ideas on which modern medicine is based. Each discipline whether scientific or not has a series of basic fundamental ideas or presuppositions on which and by virtue of which it operates. For example, each religion is based on the idea that a divine creature or God is, or several are, real and actual. Taking the other extreme of practicality, the carpenter supposes that he can manipulate his materials—the wood, nails, saw, hammer, and so on—and that he can produce some object, whether a cabinet or a house, by his operations. Other examples of presuppositions or fundamental ideas come readily to mind; our task was not to discover these in many fields of activity but to delineate those which seem proper for Medicine, to determine their significance and to discover which implications and suggestions they may contain for the discipline.

The practice of medicine would be impracticable and nearly impossible if we did not believe: that abnormal conditions can be recognized in the human body; that the living organism shares with the rest of nature the properties of being orderly, understandable and analyzable; that the living organism has features of structure and function which can be examined down to the level of the individual cells and even to subcellular ultra-structure; that disease is an alteration of the body involving both structure and function even as far as the constituent molecules; that diseases exist as patterns of bodily processes or modifications of both structure and function, the identification and classification of disease processes extending down to and depending upon the molecules constituting the body; that certain diseases have specific etiologies and all diseases are caused; and, finally, that appropriate treatment can benefit the individual patient and in many cases cure the disease. We have traced the broad outlines of the fashions in which these fundamental ideas or presuppositions of Medicine have developed.

In reviewing the development of modern medicine as traced in the elaboration of its fundamental ideas, we have been able to see great progress in both the efficiency and in the care with which the patient is treated. There have been great mistakes, and sombre episodes are not infrequent in medical history—the horrendous concoctions of the pharmacopeaia of several millenia, the gallons of blood let in the name of rational therapy over an equivalent period. At the same time it is to be recognized that major victories have been won over disease; witness the near-disappearance of syphilis, of tuberculosis and of poliomyelitis in the United States within the recent past. We are well aware of the fallacy of "Post Hoc, Ergo Propter Hoc;" we know that temporal sequence does not imply causal relationships. Yet we can believe quite honestly that the advances in medicine are responsible for the subsidence of these plagues of past generations, and of many others. In many ways the history of medicine is the history of mankind in a sort of facsimile: there have been great mistakes and yet greater victories, and there *has* been substantial progress.

The past in medicine when studied tells us that many things can be accomplished without any sound foundation of either science or theory. The clinical acumen of Sydenham and of Heberden was exercised on the basis of the four humors of Hippocrates and without laboratory aid of any substantial degree. Nevertheless, these great figures could isolate particular cases from their large experience and by recognizing the common features, identify specific illnesses. Despite this, we have reason to believe that our progress in medicine since it became scientific has been greater than ever before, and our beliefs in this regard are confirmed by declining death rates and by a general extension of life expectancy at nearly every age.

It is recalled that in the 3rd century B.C. the Greeks believed that the body was made up of four elements, earth, air, fire and water, and that this theory lasted until the Middle Ages. Again it is recalled that the Chinese theory of matter up until the 20th century had the same four Greek elements, to which was added wood. In both the ancient Greek belief and the near modern Chinese belief, there was evident a general lethargy in the progress of science in general and of medicine in particular. Only with the scientific revolution of the 15th century in the West did progress in science begin, and Medicine took several centuries to catch the momentum; the corresponding progress in medicine in China has not taken place except where Western scientific colonies have been in operation.

One particular area of increasing study and attention at the present time may be called the Mind-Body relationship. What is the nature of mind, if there is one? What of the Spirit of man? Is there a Soul? What do mind, spirit and soul have to do with the body in health and in disease? These are the questions being asked specifically in the so-called psychosomatic medicine and implicitly in the discipline of Psychiatry. In this regard, Rather has an appropriate question from Voltaire, which interestingly enough was used also by Virchow in 1847:

> "Dans quels recoins de tissu cellulaire
> Sont les talens de Virgile ou d'Homer?"

"In what recesses of the cellular tissue are the talents of Virgil or of Homer?" This is one of our main problems today, the explanation of the activities of mind in terms of the body or by the development of new and more appropriate criteria.

The tendency of one who has surveyed the building-up of a discipline, as we have reviewed the history of the fundamental ideas or presuppositions of medicine, is to attempt to predict in which directions future extensions of activity may be expected. This is contrary to Hegel's oft-quoted and pessimistic statement, "The one thing one learns from history is that nobody ever learns from history." Nevertheless it seems to be possible to recognize some areas in which considerable study and probable advance are to be expected.

The scientific methods which have heretofore been most applied

84 The Fundamental Ideas of Medicine

to the disease and to the agents causing the disease will be in increasing degree employed in the study of the other half of the complex, the patient. We shall intensify the study of the living thing in health, as such, the organism which in the case of medicine is the human being. To the findings of the probings in a diversity of species which the Organismic Biologists have directed, we shall add the data derived from the intensive study which has been given to the human being. I think personally that we shall derive a definition of the organism or living thing as an "organized continuous homeostatic individual," all terms in the definition being shared by biology and by medicine. As medicine progresses in the study of the individual and of the individual patient, it will be increasingly aware of the identity of interests and methods shared by biology and by medical practice, the identity described by W. H. Welch in 1889 and emphasized anew by Paul Weiss in 1958.

It is possible that a consideration of the fundamental ideas and presuppositions of medicine will furnish adequate ammunition for those who see potential value in a reconsideration and possible recasting of the formula by which the training of doctors takes place. This is the old question of reform of the medical school curriculum in the United States, which is raised or raises itself periodically. There is no doubt that better medicine was practiced after the reforms recommended by Flexner in 1912 but there is no good proof that Flexner's fossilized formulae are the best that can be imagined. There is much sentiment and experience to the contrary. In mathematics serious questioning is being given to the sequence in which courses are taken, whether algebra needs to follow arithmetic or could possibly precede it. Similarly in linguistics there is a not inconsiderable movement to begin with the use of the language and to follow this with vocabulary and grammar, much as a person put down in a country speaking a language different from his own learns to use the new one and then is ready for the special study. It need not be pointed out that the child learns to speak long before he knows spelling, grammar and punctuation.

There is not-unbased hope that the medical curriculum may be revised, that scientific medicine which emphasizes the experimental method will at last be willing to try a variety of experiments in medical education. Some hints of possible fashions in which this could be done can be appreciated from a consideration of the fundamental ideas or presuppositions of medicine. Little reason can be found in all good sense for the separation of anatomy from physiology since both are processes, in constant change, differentiated only by rate and duration, as discussed previously (p. 36).

Finally, considering the present status of medicine, the way in which this position has been reached, and the prospects for the future, a limited number of definite conclusions seem possible.

In regard to the past we must be proud of the accomplishments of our predecessors, and grateful for the information, dedication and noble and unselfish traditions which they have handed down to us, rather than critical of their shortcomings. It is hard to believe that medicine was already old in the 5th century before the Christian era began, but Hippocrates had this to say:

> "We ought not to reject the ancient Art, as if it were not and had not been properly founded, because it did not attain accuracy in all things, but rather, since it is capable of reaching to the greatest exactitude by reasoning, to receive it and admire its discoveries, made from a state of great ignorance, and as having been well and properly made, and not from chance."

If this could be said by Hippocrates, or by one of his school, more than twenty-three centuries ago, how much more appropriate is it today?

At the same time we must not be too complacent about the state of our own information, nor pleased at all with what we think we know. Someone has said that nothing becomes a scientist less than an aura of certainty and, although it is obvious that every scientist has not heard this particular recommendation, certainty is not possessed by an honest scientist today. The late W. G. MacCallum prefaced the seventh edition of his textbook, twenty-eight years in print and representing the wisdom and experience of a great scientist, with this quotation from Goethe:

> "It is only when we know very little about a subject that we are quite sure; and with knowledge, doubt arises and grows."

About the same sentiments were expressed several centuries

before, a little more forcibly and a little less elegantly, by the Spanish Jesuit, Balthasar Gracian:

> "Hold to nothing too violently; only a fool is convinced, and every one convinced is a fool."

If further evidence were needed of the dangers of complacency, one needs only to consult the paean of Osler in 1902, as quoted by Snapper:

> "Never has the outlook for the profession been brighter. Everywhere the physician is better trained and better equipped than he was 25 years ago. Disease is understood more thoroughly, studied more carefully and treated more skillfully. The average sum of human suffering has been reduced in a way to make the angels rejoice. Diseases familiar to our fathers and grandfathers have disappeared, the death rate from others is falling to the vanishing point and public health measures have lessened the sorrows and brightened the lives of millions."

In 1900, before Osler's address, the death rate was 1,755 per 100,000 compared with 950 per 100,000 in 1960; tuberculosis was the principal cause of death, the "Captain of the Men of Death" as Osler said, syphilis was not uncommon, diphtheria epidemics with numerous fatalities occurred every winter as did those of typhoid fever every summer. Lobar pneumonia was the "old man's friend" and blood transfusions, insulin, antibiotics, the vitamins were alike unknown. As Snapper says:

> ". . . every generation of physicians has overestimated the progress made by medicine in its own time."

While the progress of our own period has been great, we must not think it too considerable, nor on any account be satisfied with it.

Our intention and resolve as concerns the future must be that we will apply the scientific methods derived in the past and those which are being and will be developed, to a better understanding of the prime concern of medicine—the patient—and to his relief and cure. By the judicious use of experimental techniques, the methods of "interrogating nature," as Crombie calls them, we can expect, in the words of Hippocrates, "Nature to disclose her secrets without harm." Looking confidently and principally to the future, we can as physicians and as scientists be proud of our being a part in a noble company in which our fundamental ideas have been developed, Hippocrates, Hunter, Vesalius, Sydenham, Boerhaave, Virchow, Lister, Galen, Celsus and many more. In their accomplishments we share, and because of what they did, we can try to do.

Biographical Notes

Adanson, Michael (1727-1806), French naturalist of Scotch descent. Worked in electricity but best known for *Familles des Plantes* (1763), opposing classificatory ideas of Linnaeus; other botanical works.

Addison, T. (1793-1860), colleague of Bright (q.v.) at Guy's Hospital. Described pernicious anemia and results of atrophy of suprarenal capsules (adrenal glands).

Adler, Alfred (1870-1937), psychiatrist. Inventor of "Inferiority Complex." Viennese pupil of Freud (q.v.), stressing organic inferiority, including sexual, as source of neurosis.

Agricola, George (1494-1555). Studied medicine in Italy; settled in Joachimstal in Bohemia near famous mines. Wrote *De re Metallica*, published in 1553, beginning modern mineralogy, translated by U. S. president-engineer, Herbert Hoover. Agricola reintroduced ventilation into mines, lost since Roman times.

Alcmaeon of Croton (about 500 B.C.), Pythagorean; founder of experimental psychology. Dissected and vivisected animals. Discovered optic nerve; tongue, as organ of taste. Brain described as central organ of mind. Disease caused by dominance of one or several of following: heat, cold, moisture, dryness, acidity, sweetness, etc., as Anaximander's opposites, while health is balance.

Anaximander (c. 611-547), Ionian from Miletus. Taught that world was made from earth, air, fire, water, and that life began in sea and man was descended from fish.

Aquinas, St. Thomas (1225-1274), Italian, Dominican. Student of Albertus Magnus (1206-1280) who introduced him to Aristotle's philosophy. Aquinas produced system coordinating Christian belief with Hellenic philosophy, especially Aristotle's. Greatest of scholastic philosophers.

Archimedes (287-212 B.C.), greatest engineer of antiquity. Visitor to Alexandria and Egypt; discoverer of concept of Specific Gravity;

inventor of many machines including screw-pump for raising water, planetarium, and engines used in defense of his native Syracuse against Romans. Great mathematician.

Aristotle (384-322 B.C.). Born in Stagira (hence called Stagirite), colony of Greece; father was physician to King of Macedonia. Studied with Plato (q.v.) at Athens; after 20 years left, and in 342 became tutor to Alexander the Great. Returned to Athens in 335, where founded Lycaeum and taught until death of Alexander, 323. Well known as philosopher, but at best as naturalist. Founded comparative anatomy, embryology; used observation and experiment. Systems of motion and cosmology influential for centuries. Believed life depended on possession of soul or life principle; therefore, Vitalist (vita = soul). Introduced terms aorta, cetacea, etc.

Auenbrugger, L. (1722-1809). Musician, son of innkeeper, chief physician of Spanish Hospital, Vienna. Applied percussion to examination of chest (1754), dullness of sound or resonance indicating underlying disease or health. Book *Inventum novum ex percussions thoracis* published 1761, same year as Morgagni's (q.v.) *De Sedibus.*

Augustine, St. (354-430). Died as Bishop of Hippo in North Africa. Convert to Catholicism in which main accomplishments were 1) promoting knowledge and intellectuality as theologically respectable, and 2) transmission of Neoplatonism which he incorporated into Christian faith. Considered roles of science and religion; said, "the truth, wherever it is found, must be avidly seized."

Bacon, Francis (1561-1626), courtier, philosopher, prophet of science. Influential books, *Advancement of Learning* (1605) and *Novum Organum* (1620), set out a method of investigating nature and, in criticizing scholastic philosophy, widened breach of emerging sciences from predecessors. Stimulus to much later scientific work and workers recognizable.

von Baer, Karl Ernst (1792-1876), early German embryologist. Discovered human ovum. Suggested possibility of evolution of living species.

Baillie, Matthew (1761-1823). Native Scot who followed his uncles, the Hunters, to London. Worked with William Hunter and published (1795) *Morbid Anatomy,* systemically describing and illustrating disease in various organs.

Baker, George (1722-1809). Associated lead poisoning with Devonshire Colic (1767) from drinking cider contaminated with lead; isolated lead from the cider.

Bassi, Agostino (1773-1856). Amateur microscopist, showed a disease of silkworms in Italy was caused by microorganism (1836), in fact a fungus. Thus preceded Pasteur (q.v.) in study of disease caused by living agents.

Benivieni, A. (1440-1502). Florentine surgeon. Book (*de Abditis*) of 54 pages of autopsies, "only work of pathology owing nothing to anyone," published (1507) posthumously by brother.

von Bergmann, E. (1836-1907), prominent German surgeon who introduced (1886) asepsis into surgery, replacing antiseptic period of Lister (q.v.).

Bernard, Claude (1813-1878), great French physiologist and philosopher of science. His *Lectures on Experimental Medicine* range widely, discussing fundamental problems of observation, hypothesis and experiment. Investigator of liver, glycogen, digestion, blood vessel controls, etc., etc. Contributed idea of "Internal Environment" in which body cells live and on whose constancy life depends.

Bichat, M.-F.-X. (1771-1802). French histologist. Died of a wound infection contracted during dissection. Described (1801) 21 different tissues recognizable grossly, including their anatomy, physiology and pathology. Disliked microscope.

Bigelow, H. J. (1818-1890), Boston surgeon. Attendant at operation performed at Massachusetts General Hospital, using ether as anaesthetic; published account (1846, in Boston Medical and Surgical Journal).

Billroth, C. A. T. (1829-1894), Professor of Surgery at Zurich and Vienna. Devised many operations, published many papers and important book, *Surgical Pathology and Therapy* (1863). An accomplished musician and a great friend of Johannes Brahms.

Boerhaave, H. (1668-1738), Leyden physician and chemist. *Elements of Chemistry* (1724) written as text for students. *Institutiones medicae* (1708), standard physiology for a century, sought explanation of body activities in physical and chemical terms. Influenced Austrian, Scottish, English and American medicine by his pupils and theirs. Knew contemporary languages and both Hebrew and Chaldean. Music lover and amateur musician.

Böhme, J. (1575-1624), mystic, German cobbler-philosopher. Follower of Paracelsus (q.v.), Böhme thought of man as microcosm; considered man as result of development.

Bonet or Bonetus, Th. (1620-1689). Swiss physician, author of *Sepulchretum* (1679), second great book of Pathology after Benivieni and before Morgagni, encyclopedic survey of autopsy findings recorded since ancient times; over 3,000 protocols.

Bouillaud, J.-B. (1766-1881), French physician. Related heart disease to rheumatism (rheumatic fever). Active blood-letter, but most able diagnostician.

Boyle, R. (1627-1691), English chemist. Established law of relation of volume of gas to pressure. Described chemical element. Prominent in upsurge of English science, admirer of Bacon (q.v.), founder of Royal Society, London.

Brahe, T. (1546-1601), Danish astronomer. Provided by King with observatory. Later moved to Prague. Made many accurate observations of stars, moon and sun, collecting enormous mass of data, almost overwhelming his associate Kepler (q.v.).

Bright, R. (1789-1858), great physician of Guy's Hospital, London. Acute observer and clinician who noted association of kidney disease, scanty urine, dropsy; hence, Bright's Disease.

Celsus (A.D. 30). Wrote best general medical treatise in ancient Rome. His book *On Medicine* now thought to be translation with omissions, of the Greek work of a Sicilian, Titus Aufidius. High level, in best Hippocratic tradition of care and study of patients.

Charcot, J.-M. (1825-1893), French neurologist and pathologist. Best known for studies on nervous system but wrote also on kidney disease and on diseases of old age.

Chrysoloras, M. (1355-1415), Byzantine Greek. Came to Florence in 1396 as professor of Greek at University. Symmonds says, "This engagement secured the future of Greek erudition in Europe." Numerous and famous pupils, credited with stimulating many advances of Renaissance.

Cicero, M. T. (106-43 B.C.), renowned Roman orator. Author of *De Natura Deorum*, summarizing ancient viewpoints on purpose (teleology) in structure, originating with Aristotle.

Cohn, F. J. (1828-1898), eminent German botanist. Became interested in developing Bacteriology. Classified organisms, recognized spores in anthrax, supported Koch (q.v.) in presentation of studies to scientists.

Copernicus, N. (1473-1543). Versatile Polish churchman of genius; known for heliocentric view of universe, published in book just before his death, *De Revolutionibus Orbium Coelestium*. Thought of celestial motion as circular. His theory replaced Ptolemy's (q.v.) and was part of intellectual revolution of Renaissance, weakening man's belief in authorities and older teachings.

Corvisart, J.-N. (1755-1821), French cardiologist. Teacher of Laennec and Cuvier. Revived Auenbrugger's neglected percussion (1808).

Cullen, W. (1712-1790), Scottish physician, pupil of Boerhaave and teacher of William Hunter. Introduced clinical teaching methods in England.

Cushing, Harvey (1869-1939), outstanding American neurosurgeon; Harvard, Hopkins, Yale. Student of pituitary disease, medical historian.

Cuvier, G. (1769-1832), French comparative anatomist. Believed function determined form of organs. Taught fixation of basic species, catastrophic history of world, classification of current and extinct forms of life. Active controversialist.

Darwin, Charles (1809-1882). Son of physician, led by study of fossils to belief that present animal species developed from common ancestors. Voyage on *Beagle*, 1831-1836, to South America and Pacific islands convinced him of species variations. Later studied breeding of domesticated plants and animals and reviewed data from voyage from which he derived principle of selection by survival of fittest. Published, with Wallace who discovered identical theory independently, papers in 1858. Book by Darwin (1859), *Origin of Species*, describes natural selection. In 1871 published *Descent of Man*. Both works manifest influence of current philosophic ideas of progress of Spencer.

Democritus (c. 470-370 B.C.), Greek philosopher who proposed that all matter was made up of atoms (Gr., indivisible) and the void. Revival of interest in atoms in 19th century led to revival of Democritus' theory. Also stated principles of conservation of matter, the orderly nature of the observable world, and the role of sense perception in observation.

Descartes, René (1596-1650), influential French philosopher. Lived and worked in Holland. Book, *Discourse on Method* (1637), emphasized use of mathematics and deduction in study of nature, and described results of his use of these methods. His *Principles of Philosophy* (1644) emphasized and elaborated his world view derived from his methods. Neglected experimentation. System of philosophy called Cartesian, described by Liebnitz as "ante-room of true philosophy." Mechanistic viewpoint proposed by Descartes as theory, extended by disciples to mechanistic materialism.

Dioscorides (1st century A.D.). Roman army physician from Asia Minor, wrote *Materia Medica*, described and illustrated both drugs and plants from which they originated. Most influential pharmacopeia, used by Arabs and through Middle Ages into Renaissance, though unscientific and mere compendium.

Drake, D. (1785-1852), pioneering American physician and teacher. Founded medical schools in Ohio. *Essays on Medical Education* called by Garrison, "Far and away, the most important contributions ever made to the subject in this country." Original, eloquent, versatile, intellectual, poet: one of the more imposing and appealing figures in medical history.

Dutrochet, R.-J.-H. (1776-1874), French biologist who anticipated both Schleiden and Schwann in emphasizing importance of cells but whose priority has been overlooked.

Empedocles of Sicily (c. 493-433). Greek philosopher and scientist who "strove for mastery over nature." Demonstrated experimentally reality of air by inverting hollow cylinder into water; beginning of study of nature. Recognized fossils; proposed theory of stages of creation with initial imperfect forms produced.

Erasistratus (c. 275 B.C.), Alexandrian physiologist and anatomist. Observer, experimentalist, theoretician. An atomist and follower of Democritus.

Euclid (c. 330-260 B.C.). Foremost Greek mathematician of Alexandria; details of life speculative but remaining works, notably *Geometry*, most important, and standard teaching form until present century.

Eudoxus (409-356 B.C.), disciple of Plato. Made mathematical construction to support his master's viewpoints of Universe. Theorized heavenly bodies move in concentric spherical courses with earth at center. Estimated length of solar year at 365 days, 6 hours.

Fabricius ab **Aquapendente** (1533-1619), student of Fallopius at Padua. Professor of surgery (1565), taught anatomy, described development of fetus and chick embryo, valves of veins; teacher of William Harvey (q.v.).

Fallopius, G. (1523-1562), Italian anatomist, pupil of Vesalius, teacher of Fabricius. Thorough dissector, stimulating teacher, contributor to Anatomy of several structures named after him, notably fallopian tubes.

Fernel, J. (1497-1558), French physician and physiologist. Treated body functions in line with Galen's viewpoints. An observer and philosopher. Called greatest French physician of Renaissance; wrote copiously and made original descriptions.

Flexner, A. (1886-1959), American educator. Critical report on *Medical Education in the United States and Canada* (1910) stimulated restudy of subject, led to specific standards being set up, to be followed by medical schools.

da Foligno, Gentile (d. 1348). Quoted by Crombie (1. c.). Wrote *Consilium* on plague, the Black Death of the 14th century; spoke therein of "seeds (*semina*) of disease" and of *reliquae*, or infectious materials, left by patients.

Foster, Michael (1836-1907), British physiologist, embryologist. Founder of Cambridge School of Physiologists. *History of Physiology* (1901), standard sourcebook.

Fracastoro (1483-1553), Veronese physician. His idea of contagion can be blamed on his belief in 1) the atomic theory of Democritus, and 2) the theory of Paracelsus that diseases had separate existences. Thought that disease was then conveyed as small particles.

Freud, S. (1856-1939), famous Viennese psychiatrist. Pupil of Charcot. Inventor of psychoanalysis and many terms used widely in describing personality relationships. Modern influence great, both in psychiatry and beyond Freud's own field.

Funk, C. (1884-   ), Polish chemist. Found yeast cured beri-beri quite as well as rice husks. Developed concept of deficiency diseases (1912) and introduced term *vitamine*.

Galen (131-201). Native of Pergamus in Asia Minor. Early, physician to gladiators in his native city, later to Emperors Marcus Aurelius and L. Verus in Rome. Fled Rome during Plague but returned and resumed lucrative practice. Excellent clinician, clear and prolific author, Galen's views on medicine and physiology prevailed until time of Harvey (q.v.) and after. Eighty-three of his one hundred thirty-one medical works still extant. Strongly teleologic in tone, examining purpose in every situation, Galen was yet a first-class clinician—able to diagnose, willing to treat—the story of physicians for many centuries.

Galileo Galilei (1564-1642), Italian scientist, maker of the modern scientific world. Overthrew Aristotlean mechanics and concept of universe as world-centered. Versatile, working on several projects at one time, lucid author, Galileo did more to shape subsequent thinking than any other man of his time. Contrived telescope to examine the sun, moon and stars and devised microscope with which ant was studied. Forced by a faction within church to cease teaching the heliocentric Copernican theory, Galileo spent his final years in seclusion studying and writing. His *Dialogue concerning Two World Systems* (1630) is noteworthy in that the proponent of the Copernican system has much the better of the dispute while the Aristotlean, appropriately named Simplicius, argues poorly as well as having a suspicious resemblance to one of Galileo's enemies, a prominent figure in the church.

Garrod, A. (1857-1936), British physician and chemist. His *Inborn Errors of Metabolism* (1908) and other studies placed a secure chemical basis under many important clinical conditions.

von Goethe, J. W. (1749-1832). Versatile German genius, poet, anatomist, philosopher, playwright; stimulator of much research, including embryology of skull bones; vision. Views led to *Nature Philosophy*.

Goldberger, J. (1874-1929), American nutritionist. Proved "Pellagra" in human equivalent to "Black Tongue" in dogs, both diseases noninfectious and curable by nicotinic acid.

Graves, R. J. (1796-1835), Dublin physician. Introduced continental bedside methods to Irish Medicine. Description of exophthalmic goiter (1835) attached his name to the condition.

von Haller, A. (1708-1777), eminent Swiss physiologist, pupil of Boerhaave. Studied muscular contraction and role of nerves in sensation. Proponent of preformation theory of embryogenesis, that the ovum contains all future generations as preformed miniatures.

Halsted, W. S. (1852-1922), American surgeon. First professor of surgery at Johns Hopkins (1889-1922). Developed experimental surgery, introduced local anaesthesia, rubber gloves, radical mastectomy technique for carcinoma.

Harvey, W. (1578-1657), great English physician, founder of physiology. Studied under Fabricius at Padua. Practiced and investigated in London. Demonstrated circulation of blood by experiment and observation, controverting Galen, in *De Motu Cordis et Sanguinis* 1628). Subsequent studies on development of deer and chick, *de Generatione* (1651).

Heberden, W. (1710-1801), English physician. Described angina pectoris, varicella, night blindness. His *Commentaries* (1802) described a wealth of clinical details. *Essays on Mithridatium and Theriaca* (1745) removed these ancient relics of superstition from pharmacopeia.

von Hebra, F. (1816-1880), Viennese dermatologist, pupil of Skoda and Rokitansky. Based practice on histologic study of skin, beginning scientific dermatology.

Hegel, G. W. F. (1770-1831), German philosopher. System of thought idealistic and deriving from Kant. Thought much of nature unreasonable and not understandable. Died of cholera in Berlin.

Henle, J. F. G. (1809-1885), German founder of histology. *Allgemeine Anatomie* (1841). Made many fundamental discoveries in microscopic anatomy, being ranked by Garrison in histology as equivalent to Vesalius in anatomy. Noteworthy also for *On Miasms and Contagions* (1840) which proposes a system of disease inculpating living organisms.

Heraclitus (535-475 B.C.), Ionian philosopher from Ephesus. One of the earliest, semi-legendary philosophers and observers of nature, known only by quotations and allusions by later writers. Best known for idea of flux or change, "You can not step twice into the same river."

Herodotus (485-425 B.C.), Greek historian and traveller. Gullible recounter of fantastic tales but only source for much knowledge of ancient world.

Herophilus (c. 300 B.C.), Alexandrian anatomist, contemporary of Euclid. Said to have dissected human body publicly; compared human anatomy to that of animals. Separated arteries from veins by pulsation of former.

Hippocrates of Cos (460-377 B.C.), Great physician and teacher, the model for physicians to modern times. Developed the "Hippocratic method" of observation and induction; applied Greek ideas of order in external world and of cause and effect to study of disease. Many works of Hippocrates and his school transmitted as Hippocratic Corpus to modern times, serving as guide in diagnosis and prognosis over intervening centuries.

Hodgkin, T. (1798-1866), English Quaker pathologist. Worked at Guy's and described diseases of lymphoid system, including variety now associated with his name. Eccentric, independent.

von Holbach, Baron (1731-1789), philosopher. Published *Systems de la Nature* (1770) under name of Mirabaud, dead 10 years. Nothing exists but matter and motion; nature is the sum of all that exists; no purpose, no order exists, only necessity. Mechanistic materialism as logical development of Descartes.

Holmes, O. W. (1809-1894), Boston anatomist and physician. Gifted author. Paper *On the Contagiousness of Puerperal Fever* (1843) demonstrated origin of the then prevalent illness of women after delivery to be the physicians in attendance who might come directly from the autopsy room.

Homer (c. 800 B.C.), epic poet. Source of our knowledge of early Greek beliefs on life, soul, disease, etc.

Hooke, R. C. (1635-1703), versatile English scientist. Founding member of Royal Society and longtime secretary. Saw plant cells (*Micrographia*, 1665) with compound microscope.

Hume, D. (1711-1776), Scottish philosopher. Re-examined bases for beliefs, introduced idea of "process." In part, remarkable Scot was responsible for flourishing of intellectual activity in 18th century.

Hunter, John (1728-1793), Scottish surgeon, investigator and founder of experimental surgery and of comparative anatomy. Inferior school-boy, frequent truant, sent to brother, William, in London and took fire. Among many remarkable achievements was Museum, personal dissection and demonstration of over 500 species of animals. Stimulated Jenner.

Hunter, William (1718-1783), Scottish anatomist, surgeon and obstetrician. Trained at Glasgow three years with Cullen, became leading consultant and teacher in London. Trained brother, John Hunter. Greatest works, *Anatomy of Human Gravid Uterus* (1774) and demonstration of separate fetal and maternal circulations.

Isidore of Seville (560-636). Bishop whose *Etymologies,* compendium of fact and fancy arranged alphabetically and by derivations of terms, ranged from astronomy to medicine, was popular as source of knowledge up to and in Middle Ages.

Jenner, E. (1749-1823), English country physician. Correspondent and friend of John Hunter who stimulated him to observation and experiment. Best known for cowpox inoculation as protection against smallpox. Produced hypersensitivity by repeated protein injections (1798).

Jung, C. G. (1875-1961), Swiss psychiatrist. Pupil of Freud and early collaborator but later antagonist. Believed Freud's sex-centered approach to mental disease not justified.

Kepler, J. (1571-1630), German astronomer, mystic, and mathematician. Took observations of Brahe and arranged heliocentric Copernican universe, using ellipses as courses for sun, moon, earth, and stars.

Kircher, A. (1601-1680), versatile German Jesuit and writer on microscopy. In a book published in Rome in 1658 described microscopic "worms" in decaying meat and in blood of plague patients.

Koch, R. (1843-1910), German founder of bacteriology. Pupil of Henle; proved role of anthrax bacillus in causing disease; introduced staining of bacteria including that causing tuberculosis; used solid media for cultivation; set up standards to which organism suspected of causing disease must conform.

Kraepelin, E. (1856-1927), German psychiatrist. Eminent during descriptive phase of psychiatric study, classifying mental disease and separating psychoses.

Laennec, R.-T.-H. (1781-1826). French physician. Killed by tuberculosis at an early age. Inventor of stethoscope, *Traite de l'auscultation* *mediate* (1819) popularized it as diagnostic tool. Clinical-pathologic correlations of high and permanent value, cirrhosis of liver, pneumonia, peritonitis, etc., etc.

Lamarck, J.-B. (1744-1829), French biologist. Trained by Jesuits for Church but went into army, then trade, then botany, finally zoology. Classified invertebrates and, seeing apparent gradations, suggested evolution from ancestral forms. *Zoological Philosophy* (1809) described theory of evolution and suggested inheritance of acquired characters as mechanism.

de La Mettrie, J. O. (1709-1751), French physician and Cartesian philosopher. *Natural History of the Soul* (1745) brought about expulsion from France; *L'Homme Machine* (1748), expulsion from Holland. Died while personal physician and "Court Atheist" to Frederick the Great of Prussia, after self-treatment for indigestion.

Lavoisier, A. (1743-1794), French chemist. Demonstrated role of oxygen in combustion, proposed renovation of chemical theory, introduced modern name of many chemical substances. Founder of modern chemistry. Guillotined with famous phrase, "The republic has no need of scientists," during the French Revolution because he was Tax Agent of King.

van Leeuwenhoek, A. (1632-1723), pioneer Dutch microscopist. Linen merchant of Delft who first described many living things, circulation in capillaries of tadpole tail (1688), spermatozoa (1677), plant cells, protozoa, probably bacteria. Published findings in letters to Royal Society, London.

von Leibnitz, G. W. (1646-1716), German philosopher, mathematician. Shares with Newton discovery of calculus. Postulator of *Monads* as essential units of matter, like *Atoms* of Democritus.

Lind, J. (1736-1812), Scottish naval surgeon. *Treatise on Scurvy* (1754) suggested role of deficiency in diet and recommended citrus fruits for its prevention.

Linnaeus, C. (1707-1778), Swedish physician and botanist. *System of Nature* (1735), going through twelve editions, begins classification of living things. Groupings were Classes, Orders, Genera, Species, with binomial nomenclature still in use. Classified not only animals and plants but also diseases and minerals.

Lister, Lord (1827-1912), English Quaker physician. London graduate working in Edinburgh; stimulated by Pasteur's discovery of organisms in putrefaction, attempted antiseptic surgery, reducing mortality by 66 per cent. Published, 1867, *On the Antiseptic Principle* in *Surgery*. Many other discoveries preceded and succeeded this epoch-making paper. Greatest scientific surgeon.

Livy, T. (59 B.C.-17 A.D.), Roman historian, encyclopedist. Often inaccurate compendium survived through Middle Ages as source of information and misinformation on biologic and medical subjects.

Locke, J. (1632-1704), Oxford philosopher. *Essay on Human Understanding* influential in stimulating re-examination of foundations of scientific observation.

Long, Crawford (1815-1878), Georgia physician and Pennsylvania graduate. Employed ether as anaesthetic (1842) but never published his results, having only local influence.

Lyell, C. (1797-1875), English geologist. *Principles of Geology* (1830-33) described genesis of rocks and their break-up. Book influential on Darwin, leading to early observations and in time to Evolutionary Theory.

MacCallum, W. G. (1874-1944), Canadian-born, professor of pathology at Johns Hopkins, student and successor of Welch. Discovered (1897) as medical student sexual form of malarial parasite, later role of parathyroid glands in calcium metabolism, many anatomic and histologic features of importance.

Magendie, F. (1783-1855), French physician, part-time physiologist, teacher of Claude Bernard. Did important investigations on nervous system and in other areas. Introduced experimental methods.

Maimonides, M. (1135-1204), Jewish philosopher-physician from Spain. Brought as physician to Saladin. Critical of Galen's theories. Best known work is *Guide to the Perplexed*, still highly readable and popular.

Malpighi, M. (1628-1694), Italian physician, professor. First to see (1660) the capillaries in living animal, completing circulation of Harvey. Exploited microscope as tool of study; described renal glomerulus and splenic follicles, both named after him. Caught in anti-scientific reaction of his time, rejected by his colleagues, died alone and friendless.

Mendel, G. (1822-1884), German monk and father of Genetics. Sent report of his studies to scientists, including Naegeli, but received no recognition until 1900.

Mitchell, S. Weir (1829-1914), Philadelphia neurologist and pupil of Claude Bernard. Excellent clinician, acute observer, facile and voluminous writer. Both poet and novelist.

Morgagni, G. B. (1682-1771), Italian anatomist and for fifty-six years professor at Padua. His report of autopsy findings *De Sedibus et*

Causis Morborum (1761) begins modern pathology, in comparing
postmorten appearances with clinical records.

Müller, J. (1801-1858), versatile German scientist, both histologist and
physiologist. Exceptional teacher, having Schwann, Henle, Virchow, DuBois-Reymond and Helmholtz among better known
pupils. Solid scientific contributions; few publications.

Newton, I. (1642-1727), greatest English physicist. Completed work of
Brahe, Kepler, and Galileo by hypothesizing action of gravity to
operate not only on the earth but throughout the universe. Mathematics was utilized to explain events in universe. In the Renaissance
tradition, which is that of modern science, the "How" became more
important than the "Why." Laws of Motion and Cosmology influential until present century. Recent advances in physics and elec-
tronics depend largely on departure from Newtonian Mechanics.

Nicander (2nd century B.C.), Greek physician, poet. Wrote on poisons;
classic description of lead poisoning, colic, paralysis, ocular disturbances.

Oken, L. (1779-1851), German philosopher, associate of Schelling and
member of school of *Nature-philosophers*. Book, *Elements of Physio-
Philosophy* (1810), best statement of beliefs, most influential in
biologic sciences in Germany in nineteenth century, notably in development of cell theory and cellular pathology.

Oribasius (325-400), Greek physician, called by Garrison "torch-bearer."
His predecessors' work might have been lost except for his writings;
Galen notably lauded and admired.

Osler, Sir William (1849-1919), Canadian-born physician, Professor of
Medicine at McGill, Pennsylvania, and opened Johns Hopkins with
Halsted, Welch and Kelly (The Big Four). Regius Professor of
Medicine at Oxford, 1904-1919. Scholar, teacher, classicist, historian,
admirable diagnostician and human being. Called by general con-
sent the greatest physician of his time—in tradition of Hippocrates,
Boerhaave, Heberden; bedside teacher.

Paracelsus (1493-1541), Swiss physician, teacher, alchemist. Violent
tempered, abusive controversialist, enthusiast and iconoclast. His
sincere attacks on time-honored beliefs represented and furnished
some of his skepticism characteristic of the Renaissance.

Paré, A. (1517-1590), French surgeon whose work *On Wounds* published in 1545 from military experience represents a new rationality
in surgery. Wrote epitome of *Fabrica* of Vesalius, helping to popu-
larize it. From barber's apprentice became most prominent and
popular surgeon of his time. His phrase, "I treated him, God cured

him," represents extraordinary appreciation of his role as surgeon of his time.

Parry, C. H. (1755-1822), esteemed English physician and clinician. First to describe a number of diseases, including exophthalmic goiter (1786).

Pasteur, L. (1822-1895), French savant, with Koch the founder of bacteriology. Trained originally in chemistry, led from study of forms of tartaric acid to that of the organisms acting on one of its isomers, to the yeasts of wine, to disease of silkworms, to animal diseases and, after 1880, to organisms causing human disease. Discovered principle of immunization, efficacy of antisera, etc., etc. Patient, learned, pleasant genius. Suffered "stroke" at age of 48 which left him partially paralyzed, but much of best work done despite this handicap.

Perkin, W. (1838-1907), English chemist. Founder of synthetic dye industry; discovery in 1856 of mauve dye, produced in attempt to get quinine by oxidation of aniline derivatives. When only 18, Perkin formed own company, ancestor of one of world's great firms. Aniline dyes found much use and value in the developing biologic sciences, pathology, bacteriology.

Peter of Abano (1250-1316), medieval physician, author of important and popular book *Conciliator*, analyzing features of disease. Medical textbook for students who were supposed to memorize material and repeat verbatim at examinations, a custom largely lost from medical teaching.

Pinel, P. (1745-1826), French physician. Began modern treatment of mental illnesses (1793), removing chains and manacles previously used for restraint.

Plato (427-327 B.C.), Greek philosopher, author, playwright, pupil of Socrates, Aristotle's teacher. Whitehead calls western philosophy "Commentary on Plato." Originator of concept of reality of ideas (horse, house) and non-reality of individual. System capable of teleologic and mystic development. By Alexandrian neoplatonism, Plato influenced St. Augustine and Church through middle ages. Idea of perfect shape being sphere, deriving from Pythagoreans, induced Plato to suggest concentric spheres for shape of Universe with earth at center. Pupil, Eudoxus, mathematized spherical courses of sun, moon, etc. Aristotle made spheres crystalline, transparent.

Pliny, G. P. (23-79), great Roman encyclopedist. Killed while watching too closely an eruption of Vesuvius. His *Natural History*, charmingly and circumstantially written with interesting details, while frequently inexact, is one of the great sources on ancient manners and customs as well as many other things.

Priestley, J. (1733-1804), English chemist and investigator. Improved techniques for study of gases, demonstrated green plants could renew respired air, making it again breathable. Isolated oxygen. Hampered by "obstinate adherence to the old phlogiston theory" (Singer), discoveries only properly interpreted by Lavoisier.

Pringle, J. (1707-1782), Scottish physician, pupil of Boerhaave. Later, Surgeon General of British Army. Established principles of military sanitation (1752), improved ventilation of wards, barracks and ships.

Ptolemy, C. (A.D. 100), Alexandrian astronomer, geographer. Formalized the Aristotlean earth-centered scheme of the universe, used eccentrics and epicycles to explain planetary motions, producing idea which prevailed until Copernican revolution. Geography included Malay Peninsula and China, and east and west coasts of Africa. Best preserved book of Ptolemy is his *Almagest*, the astrologic treatise used until Renaissance as aid in treatment of disease.

Purkinje, J. (1787-1869), Czech scientist. Observed (1835) nucleus in hen's egg and described animal tissues as made up of packed cells as in plants. Friend of Goethe. First physiology laboratory (in his own house) in 1824. Physiologic Institute, 1842; introduced term "protoplasm."

Pythagoras (c. 540 B.C.), Greek philosopher, mystic, by tradition founder of mathematics. Established religious brotherhood; believed to have arrived at much of geometry included in Euclid. Identified numbers with things.

Rayer, P.-F.-O. (1793-1867), French physician. Early dermatologist, basing diagnosis on pathology. Great work on kidney disease (1837-41).

Richet, C. (1850-1935), French physiologist, versatile investigator whose studies on immunity produced term "anaphylaxis," 1902.

Ricord, P. (1800-1889), American-born French physician, separated syphilis from gonorrhea by inoculations of patients. Witty, rude and source of fable.

Rokitansky, C. (1804-1878), Viennese pathologist with personal experience derived from over 30,000 autopsies. Voluminous and able writer, notable for work on diseases of arteries and on congenital malformations of the heart.

Röntgen, W. K. (1845-1923), physicist. Described x-ray in 1895. Immensely valuable in medical diagnosis, the elaboration of data based on the discovery of the x-ray has been a great stimulus in both pure and applied physics.

Rush, B. (1745-1813), Philadelphia physician, medical student of Cullen at Edinburgh. Signer of Declaration of Independence. Excellent clinician, able writer. Foremost physician of his time.

Schleiden, M. (1804-1881), Austrian botanist, proposed cell theory for plants (1838) and suggested value of plant embryology.

Schwann, T. (1810-1882), German biologist, pupil of Müller (q.v.). Cellular doctrine promulgated (1839), with nucleus, protoplasm, cell membrane described in many examples.

Semmelweiss, I. P. (1818-1865), Hungarian pupil of Skoda and Rokitansky in Vienna. Proved infection in puerperal fever (1847), that it came with the flow of students and physicians from autopsy room to the obstetric wards, and that it could be reduced 90 per cent by cleanliness. Criticized and disputed, left Vienna and died insane.

Simpson, J. Y. (1811-1870), eminent Edinburgh obstetrician-surgeon, used ether for anaesthetic in 1846, later substituting chloroform for same purpose. Foe of Lister and against antisepsis in surgery despite earlier studies showing dangers in hospital vs. home surgery.

Skoda, J. (1805-1881), Viennese physician. Therapeutic nihilist, impressive diagnostician and student of disease. Notable for regarding patient chiefly as object of investigation.

Smith, Theobald (1859-1934), American experimental pathologist and immunologist. Demonstrated immunization by bacterial products (1886); anaphylaxis (1903); separated human and bovine types of tubercle bacillus (1898).

Socrates (469-399 B.C.), Greek philosopher who turned attention of philosophy away from study of nature to a concern for personal and religious problems—Self, Soul. Major figure in history of Thought, teacher of Plato.

Spencer, H. (1820-1903), British philosopher who in 1852, before Darwin's publications, described progress as caused by survival of adaptable forms. After Darwin's *Origin of Species* (1859), Spencer extended idea of "survival of fittest" to society and to nations; free trade and economic competition related to struggle for survival.

Spinoza, B. (1632-1677), Dutch philosopher of Jewish extraction. Earned living as lens-grinder. System of *Ethics*, his most famous work, derives from axioms and definitions like Euclid's geometry.

Strato (c. 300 B.C.), first head of Alexandrian museum, pupil of Theophrastus who was best pupil of Aristotle. Experimentalist and acute observer, instituted Aristotlean methods of study in Museum.

Sydenham, T. (1624-1689). Educated at Oxford and Montpelier; Puritan cavalry officer. Excellent clinician, revolted against theorizing and experimentation. Interest in epidemiology; excellent descriptions of diseases and illnesses.

Sylvius, F. (1614-1672), Leyden physician and physiologist, bedside teacher; Willis and Stensen among his pupils. Chemical studies on digestion, saliva, pancreatic juice, acids and bases.

Thales (c. 600 B.C.), semi-legendary Ionian philosopher of Greek descent. Practical man, said to have developed method for measuring distance of ships at sea and other aids to investigation; prediction of eclipse later untrue addition to fame. First proposed theory of nature of matter.

Theophrastus (372-287 B.C.), pupil of Aristotle. Founder of Botany as special area of study, knew 500 species of plants. Teacher of Strato (q.v.).

Trousseau, A. (1801-1867), eminent French physician, originator of modern use of tracheotomy, thoracentesis, intubation. Great teacher, author of standard medical work of his time.

Van Beneden, E. (1845-1910), Belgian biologist. Great contributor to knowledge of chromosomes, their number, halving in maturation of sex-cells, meiosis, etc.

Vesalius, A. (1514-1564), great anatomist, outstanding medical figure between Galen and Harvey. Made anatomy into scientific discipline with *De Fabrica Humani Corporis* (1543), with illustrations by Calcar of superior quality. Gave up Anatomy and became court physician to Charles V. Died during return from pilgrimage to Jerusalem.

Virchow, R. (1821-1902), great German pathologist, introducer of Cellular Pathology (1858). Student of Müller (q.v.). Professor of Pathology at Berlin (1856); politician; epidemiologist; anthropologist; editor; author; superb in all these areas. Described many features of disease for the first time; active controversialist. When shown bones of Neanderthal man (1857), decided they were example of arthritis; opposed Darwinian theory of evolution.

Vitruvius (c. 50 B.C.-20 A.D.), Roman engineer. Book *On Architecture* in ten volumes, compendium of then current practice and experience of past. Historical value of work considerable as it concerns Greek science. Chapter on Decadence in Fresco Painting!

Voltaire (1694-1778), born Arouet, was French philosopher of Enlightenment, Political exile for time in England, returned to France with admiration for Locke and Newton. Stimulated translation of works into French, influencing thought of time. Many-sided genius; novelist, poet. Advocate of unpopular causes; fierce controversialist.

Welch, W. H. (1850-1934), American pathologist of distinction. Student of Weigert and Cohnheim; teacher of many pathology professors, as Professor at Johns Hopkins (1884-1916). Later Director of School of Hygiene (1916-26), Institute of History of Medicine (1926-30). Articulate writer on subjects as diverse as medical education, biology in relation to medicine, medical research, antivivisection.

Wells, H. (1815-1848), Hartford dentist, used nitrous oxide as anaesthetic in tooth extraction (1845). Later a patient died under nitrous oxide and Wells committed suicide.

Withering, W. (1741-1799), able English clinician, most notable for introduction of digitalis (as foxglove) in dropsy (1776). Said to have been told of medicinal value of the plant by country woman.

Wunderlich, C. R. A. (1815-1877), German physician. Many contributions but greatest was clinical thermometry. Until his treatise (1868), fever had been treated as a disease.

References and Suggestions for Additional Reading

The number in parentheses following each citation refers to which of the following categories the article or book most directly relates.

1. History of Medicine.
2. History of Science.
3. History of Philosophy.

4. History in General.
5. Philosophy of Science.
6. Current Biologic Thought.

7. Miscellaneous.

AGAR, W. E.: *A Contribution to the Theory of the Living Organism.* Melbourne, University Press, 1951. (6)

BAKER, J. R.: The cell theory: a restatement and critique. *Quart. J. Micr. Sci.*, 90:87, 1949. (2)

BECKNER, M.: *The Biological Way of Thought.* New York, Columbia University, 1959. (6)

VON BERTALANFFY, LUDWIG: *Problems of Life.* New York, Harper, 1960. (6)

BETTMANN, OTTO L.: *A Pictorial History of Medicine.* Springfield, Thomas, 1962. (1)

BLIN-STOYLE, R. J. *et al.*: *Turning Points in Physics.* Amsterdam, North-Holland, 1960. (2)

BONNER, JOHN T.: *The Ideas of Biology.* New York, Harper, 1926. (5)

BOYD, WILLIAM: *Pathology for the Physician.* Philadelphia, Lea and Febiger, 1958. (7)

BRONOWSKI, J.: *The Common Sense of Science.* London, Spottiswoode, 1960. (5)

BROOKS, CHANDLER McC., and CRANEFIELD, PAUL F., editors: *The Historical Development of Physiological Thought.* New York, Hafner, 1959. (2)

BULLOCK, WILLIAM: *The History of Bacteriology.* London, Oxford University, 1938. (2)

BURGH, W. G.: *The Legacy of the Ancient World.* Baltimore, Penguin, 1961. (4)

BURTT, EDWIN A.: *The Metaphysical Foundations of Modern Physical Science.* New York, Doubleday, 1954. (5)

BURY, J. B.: *The Idea of Progress: Inquiry into Its Origin and Growth.* New York, Columbia University, 1932. (5)

BUTTERFIELD, H.: *The Origins of Modern Science, 1300-1800.* New York, Macmillan, 1960. (2)

CASSIRER, ERNST: *The Philosophy of the Enlightenment.* Boston, Beacon, 1960. (3)

CLARK, G. N.: *Science and Social Welfare in the Age of Newton.* Oxford, Clarendon, 1949. (2)

COLLINGWOOD, R. G.: *The Idea of History.* New York, Oxford University, 1956. (4)

COLLINGWOOD, R. G.: *The Idea of Nature.* New York, Oxford University, 1960. (2)

CORNFORD, FRANCIS: *Before and After Socrates.* Cambridge, University Press, 1960. (3)

CROMBIE, A. C.: Galileo's conception of scientific truth, literature and science, *Proceedings of the Sixth Triennial Congress.* Oxford, Blackwell, 1955. (2)

CROMBIE, A. C.: *Augustine to Galileo.* London, Mercury, 1961. (2)

DAMPIER, SIR WILLIAM: *A History of Science and Its Relations with Philosophy and Religion.* New York, Macmillan, 1938. (2)

DANTO, ARTHUR, and MORGENBESSER, SIDNEY: *Philosophy of Science.* New York, Meridian, 1960. (5)

ERDMANN, J. E.: *A History of Philosophy* (trans. by W. S. Hough). New York, Macmillan, 1890. (3)

FARRINGTON, BENJAMIN: *Greek Science.* London, Penguin, 1953. (2)

FERM, VERGILIUS, editor: *A History of Philosophical Systems.* Ames, Littlefield, 1958. (3)

FLOREY, H.: *General Pathology.* Philadelphia, Saunders, 1962. (7)

FOLLIS, R. H., JR.: Cellular pathology and the development of the deficiency disease concept, *Bull. Hist. Med., 34*:291, 1960. (1)

FRAKE, CHARLES O.: The diagnosis of disease among the subanun of Mindanao, *Stanford Med. Bull., 19*:105, August, 1961. (7)

FRANK, PHILIPP, editor: *The Validation of Scientific Theories.* New York, Collier, 1961. (5)

FRANK, PHILIPP: *Philosophy of Science.* Englewood Cliffs, Prentice-Hall, 1962. (5)

FRANKFORT, H., and H. A., WILSON, JOHN A., and JACOBSEN, THORKILD: *Before Philosophy.* Baltimore, Penguin, 1959. (3)

GARRISON, FIELDING H.: *An Introduction to the History of Medicine.* Philadelphia, Saunders, 1960. (1)

GILBY, THOMAS: *St. Thomas Aquinas, Philosophical Texts.* New York, Oxford University, 1960. (3)

GOODFIELD, G. J.: *The Growth of Scientific Physiology.* London, Hutchinson, 1960. (2)

GUTHRIE, D.: *A History of Medicine.* Philadelphia, Lippincott, 1946. (1)

HALDANE, J. B. S.: *The Philosophical Basis of Biology.* London, Hodder and Stoughton, 1931. (6)

HALL, A. R.: *The Scientific Revolution.* Boston, Beacon, 1957. (2)

HARRISON, T. R. *et al.: Principles of Internal Medicine.* New York, Blakiston, 1954. (7)

HENDERSON, L. J.: *The Order of Nature; An Essay.* Cambridge, Harvard University, 1917 (6)

HITTI, PHILIP K.: *The Arabs.* Princeton, Princeton University, 1949. (4)

HÖFFDING, HARALD: *A History of Modern Philosophy.* Volumes I and II. London, Dover, 1955. (3)

HOOK, SIDNEY: *Dimensions of Mind.* New York, Collier, 1961. (5)

HULL, L. W. H.: *History and Philosophy of Science,* London, Longmans, 1959. (2)

JOHNSTONE, J.: *Philosophy of Biology,* Cambridge, University Press, 1914. (5)

KEMENY, JOHN G.: *A Philosopher Looks at Science.* Princeton, D. Van Nostrand, 1959. (5)

LINDSAY, JEAN, editor: *A Short History of Science.* New York, Doubleday, 1959. (2)

LONG, E. R.: *A History of Pathology.* Baltimore, Williams and Wilkins, 1928. (2)

LOVEJOY, ARTHUR O.: *Essays in the History of Ideas.* New York, Putnam's, 1960. (7)

LOVEJOY, ARTHUR O.: *The Great Chain of Being.* New York, Harper, 1960. (2)

MADDEN, EDWARD H.: *The Structure of Scientific Thought.* Boston, Houghton Mifflin, 1960. (5)

McMANUS, J. F. A.: Rudolf Virchow in 1858, *Lab. Invest.,* 7:549, 1958. (1)

MAINX, F.: Foundations of biology, *Internat. Ency. Unified Science,* Volume 1, #9. Chicago, University of Chicago, 1955. (6)

MAJOR, RALPH H.: *Classic Descriptions of Disease.* Springfield, Thomas, 1945. (1)

MAJOR, RALPH H.: *A History of Medicine*. Springfield, Thomas, 1954. (1)

MASON, S. F.: *Main Currents of Scientific Thought*. New York, Abelard-Schuman, 1956. (2)

MEDAWAR, P. B.: *The Uniqueness of the Individual*. London, Methuen, 1957. (6)

METTLER, CECILIA C.: *History of Medicine*. Philadelphia, Blakiston, 1947. (1)

MULLER, HERBERT J.: *Science and Criticism*. New Haven, Yale University, 1944. (6)

MULLER, HERBERT J.: *The Loom of History*. New York, Harper, 1958. (4)

NEUGEBAUER, O.: *The Exact Sciences in Antiquity*. Copenhagen, Princeton University, 1957. (2)

ONIANS, RICHARD B.: *The Origins of European Thought*. Cambridge, University Press, 1954. (7)

PLAUT, A.: Virchow's "cellular pathology" in the framework of biology and medicine, *J. Washington Acad. Sci.*, 50:1, 1960. (2)

PLEDGE, H. T.: *Science Since 1500*. New York, Harper, 1959. (2)

RACKHAM, H. (trans.): *Cicero's de Natura Deorum*. New York, Putnam's, 1933. (7)

RADHAKRISHN, S.: *History of Philosophy, Eastern and Western*. London, Geo. Allen and Unwin, 1953. (3)

RADIN, PAUL: *Primitive Man as Philosopher*. New York, Dover, 1957. (7)

RADEL, EMMANUEL: *The History of Biological Theories*, translated by E. J. Hatfield. New York, Oxford University, 1930. (2)

RATHER, L. J.: The disease entity, *Stanford Med. Bull.*, 19:142, August, 1961. (1)

ROWSE, A. L.: *The Uses of History*. London, Hodder & Stoughton, 1946. (4)

RUSSELL, E. S.: *The Directiveness of Organic Activities*. Cambridge, University Press, 1946. (6)

DE SANTILLANA, GIORGIO: *The Origins of Scientific Thought*. New York, Mentor, 1961. (2)

SARTON, GEORGE: *Ancient Science and Modern Civilization*. New York, Harper, 1959. (2)

SARTON, GEORGE: *The Life of Science*. Bloomington, Indiana University, 1960. (2)

SCHRODINGER, ERWIN: *What is Life?* New York, Doubleday, 1944. (5)

References and Suggestions for Additional Reading 111

SHERRINGTON, SIR CHARLES: *Man on His Nature.* New York, Doubleday, 1953. (5)
SIGERIST, HENRY E.: *A History of Medicine,* Volume I. New York, Oxford University, 1951. (1)
SIGERIST, HENRY E.: *A History of Medicine,* Volume II, edited by Ludwig Edelstein. New York, Oxford University, 1961. (1)
SINGER, CHARLES: *A Short History of Scientific Ideas to 1900.* Oxford, Clarendon, 1959. (2)
SINNOTT EDMUND W.: *Cell and Psyche: The Biology of Purpose.* New York, Harper Torchbook, 1961. (6)
SINNOTT, EDMUND W.: *Matter, Mind and Man.* New York, Atheneum, 1962. (6)
SNAPPER, I.: *Meditations on Medicine and Medical Education.* New York, Grune & Stratton, 1956. (1)
SOMMERHOFF, P.: *Analytical Biology.* London, Oxford University, 1950. (6)
SYMONDS, JOHN A.: *The Revival of Learning.* New York, Putnam's, 1960. (4)
TOULMIN, STEPHEN: *The Philosophy of Science.* London, Hutchinson, 1960. (5)
WADDINGTON, C. H.: *Biological Organization, Cellular and Subcellular (UNESCO Conference).* London, New York, Pergamon, 1959. (6)
WARTMAN, WILLIAM B.: *Medical Teaching in Western Civilization.* Chicago, Year Book, 1961. (1)
WEISS, P.: The cell in development, *Lab. Invest.,* 8:415, 1959. (6)
WHEELER, W. M.: *Essays in Philosophical Biology.* Cambridge, Harvard University, 1939. (6)
WHITEHEAD, ALFRED N.: *Science and the Modern World.* New York, Mentor, 1959. (3)
WIENER, N.: *Cybernetics.* New York, Wiley and Sons, 1948.
WIGHTMAN, WILLIAM P.: *The Growth of Scientific Ideas.* New Haven, Yale University, 1953. (2)
WILLEY, BASIL: *The Eighteenth Century Background.* London, Chatto and Windus, 1953. (4)
WILLEY, BASIL: *The Seventeenth Century Background.* New York, Doubleday, 1953. (4)
WILLIAMS, R.: *Biochemical Individuality.* New York, Wiley, 1956. (7)
WOLF, A.: *A History of Science, Technology, & Philosophy in the 18th Century.* New York, Harper, 1961. (2)
WOODGER, J. H.: *Biological Principles.* London, Kegan Paul, 1929. (6)

WRIGHT, G. PAYLING: *An Introduction to Pathology.* New York, Longman, Green & Co., 1958.
WYNN-REEVES, JOAN: *Body and Mind in Western Thought.* New York, Penguin, 1956.

Index

(Biographical Notes are arranged alphabetically beginning on page 89.)